Use of Neuroleptics in Children

Clinical Practice

Number 37

Judith H. Gold, M.D., F.R.C.P.C.
Elissa P. Benedek, M.D.
Series Editors

Use of Neuroleptics in Children

Edited by

Mary Ann Richardson, Ph.D.
Gary Haugland, M.A.

American Psychiatric Press, Inc.
Washington, DC
London, England

Note: The authors have worked to ensure that all information in this book concerning drug dosages, schedules, and routes of administration is accurate as of the time of publication and consistent with standards set by the U.S. Food and Drug Administration and the general medical community. As medical research and practice advance, however, therapeutic standards may change. For this reason and because human and mechanical errors sometimes occur, we recommend that readers follow the advice of a physician who is directly involved in their care or the care of a member of their family.

Manufactured in the United States of America on acid-free paper
First Edition 99 98 97 96 4 3 2 1

American Psychiatric Press, Inc.
1400 K Street, N.W., Washington, DC 20005

Library of Congress Cataloging-in-Publication Data
Use of neuroleptics in children / edited by Mary Ann Richardson and Gary Haugland. — 1st ed.
p. cm. — (Clinical practice series ; 37)
Includes bibliographical references and index.
ISBN 0-88048-475-6 (alk. paper)
1. Antipsychotic drugs. 2. Pediatric psychopharmacology.
I. Richardson, Mary Ann. II. Haugland, Gary, 1947– .
III. Series: Clinical practice ; no. 37.
[DNLM: 1. Antipsychotic Agents—therapeutic use.
2. Psychopharmacology—in infancy & childhood. W1 CL767J no. 37
1996 / QV 77.9 U84 1996]
RJ504.7.U84 1996
6182.92'8918—dc20
DNLM/DLC
for Library of Congress 95-23083
CIP

British Library Cataloguing in Publication Data
A CIP record is available from the British Library.

Contents

Contributors ix

Introduction to the Clinical Practice Series xiii
Judith H. Gold, M.D., F.R.C.P.C.

Introduction xix
Mary Ann Richardson, Ph.D.
Gary Haugland, M.A.

1 Overview of Neuroleptic Use in Child Psychiatric Disorders 1
Magda Campbell, M.D.
Nilda M. Gonzalez, M.D.

2 Neuroleptic Use in Children and Adolescents Hospitalized for Psychiatric Disorders: Gender Issues and Implications 23
Julie Magno Zito, Ph.D.
Thomas J. Craig, M.D., M.P.H.
Joseph A. Wanderling, M.A.

3 Typicality and Atypicality in the Development of Neuroleptic Side Effects in Child and Adolescent Psychiatric Patients 43
Mary Ann Richardson, Ph.D.
Gary Haugland, M.A.

4 Haloperidol in Hospitalized Schizophrenic Children 67
Elizabeth Kay Spencer, M.D.
Vivian Kafantaris, M.D.
Maria V. Padron-Gayol, M.D.
Carl R. Rosenberg, Ph.D.

5 Cognitive Effects of Neuroleptic Treatment in Children With Conduct Disorder 85
Laurence L. Greenhill, M.D.
Jeffrey M. Halperin, Ph.D.
Joseph Barmack, Ph.D.

6 Stereotypies and Neuroleptic-Related Dyskinesias in Children With Autism 121
Richard P. Malone, M.D.

7 Treatment of Tic Disorders With Neuroleptic Drugs 137
Arthur K. Shapiro, M.D.
Elaine Shapiro, Ph.D.

8 Cognitive Effects of Neuroleptic Use in Children With Tourette's Syndrome 171
Floyd R. Sallee, M.D.
Christina M. Rock, B.S.
Lori A. Head, Pharm.D.

9 Neuroleptic-Induced Behavior Disorders in Patients With Tourette's Syndrome 185
Ruth Dowling Bruun, M.D.
Cathy L. Budman, M.D.

Appendix Cross-Referenced List of Selected Medications Used in This Book 199

Index 201

Contributors

Joseph Barmack, Ph.D.
Visiting Professor of Psychology, Division of Child and Adolescent Psychiatry, Columbia College of Physicians and Surgeons, New York, New York

Ruth Dowling Bruun, M.D.
Clinical Associate Professor of Psychiatry, Department of Psychiatry, Cornell University Medical College, Manhasset, New York

Cathy L. Budman, M.D.
Assistant Professor of Psychiatry, Cornell University Medical College, New York, New York; and Coordinator, Movement Disorders Center, North Shore University Hospital, Manhasset, New York

Magda Campbell, M.D.
Professor of Psychiatry, Department of Psychiatry, New York University Medical Center, New York, New York

Thomas J. Craig, M.D., M.P.H.
Professor of Psychiatry and Behavioral Science, SUNY at Stony Brook, School of Medicine, Stony Brook, New York; and Medical Director of Substance Abuse Services, Northport VA Medical Center, Northport, New York

Nilda M. Gonzalez, M.D.
Instructor in Psychiatry, New York Hospital—Cornell University Medical College, Westchester Division, White Plains, New York

Laurence L. Greenhill, M.D.
Associate Professor of Clinical Psychiatry, Division of Child and Adolescent Psychiatry, Columbia College of Physicians and Surgeons, Columbia University; Research Psychiatrist II, New York State Psychiatric Institute; and Director, Disruptive Behavior Disorders Clinic, Child Psychiatry Outpatient Unit, Columbia Presbyterian Medical Center, New York, New York

Jeffrey M. Halperin, Ph.D.
Associate Professor of Psychology, Queens College, City University of New York, Queens Village, New York

Gary Haugland, M.A.
Research Scientist, Epidemiology and Health Services Research Laboratory, Statistical Sciences and Epidemiology Division, Nathan S. Kline Institute for Psychiatric Research, Orangeburg, New York

Lori A. Head, Pharm.D.
Assistant Professor of Pharmacology and Instructor in Psychiatry, Medical University of South Carolina, Charleston, South Carolina

Vivian Kafantaris, M.D.
Assistant Physician-in-Charge, Child and Adolescent Psychiatry Ambulatory Services, Schneider Children's Hospital, Long Island Jewish Medical Center, New Hyde Park, New York

Richard P. Malone, M.D.
Director, Child and Adolescent Psychiatry Research, Hahnemann University, Department of Mental Health Sciences, Philadelphia, Pennsylvania

Maria V. Padron-Gayol, M.D.
Clinical Assistant Professor of Psychiatry, New York University Medical Center, New York, New York

Mary Ann Richardson, Ph.D.
Chief, Movement Disorders Program, Nathan S. Kline Institute for Psychiatric Research; Clinical Director, Movement Disorders Program, Rockland Psychiatric Center, Orangeburg, New York; and Research Associate Professor of Psychiatry, New York University Medical Center, New York, New York

Christina M. Rock, B.S.
Graduate Student, Department of Psychology, University of Virginia at Blacksburg, Blacksburg, Virginia

Carl R. Rosenberg, Ph.D.
Research Assistant Professor of Environmental Medicine, New York University Medical Center, New York, New York

Floyd R. Sallee, M.D.
Associate Professor of Psychiatry, Department of Psychiatry, Medical University of South Carolina, Charleston, South Carolina

Arthur K. Shapiro, M.D.
Clinical Professor of Psychiatry and Director, Tourette and Tic Laboratory and Clinic, Mount Sinai School of Medicine, New York, New York

Elaine Shapiro, Ph.D.
Associate Clinical Professor (Psychology) of Psychiatry and Co-Director, Tourette and Tic Laboratory and Clinic, Mount Sinai School of Medicine, New York, New York

Elizabeth Kay Spencer, M.D.
Research Assistant Professor of Psychiatry, New York University Medical Center, New York, New York

Joseph A. Wanderling, M.A.
Research Scientist, Nathan S. Kline Institute for Psychiatric Research, Orangeburg, New York

Julie Magno Zito, Ph.D.
Associate Professor, Department of Pharmacy Practice and Science, School of Pharmacy, University of Maryland at Baltimore, Baltimore, Maryland

Introduction
to the Clinical Practice Series

Over the years of its existence, the series of monographs entitled *Clinical Insights* has gradually become focused on providing current, factual, and theoretical material of interest to clinicians working outside of a hospital setting. To reflect this orientation, the name of the series has been changed to *Clinical Practice.*

The Clinical Practice Series will provide books that will give mental health clinicians a practical, clinical approach to a variety of psychiatric problems. These books will provide up-to-date literature reviews and emphasize the most recent treatment methods. Thus, the publications in the series should be of interest to clinicians working in both psychiatry and the other mental health professions.

Each year, a number of books in the series will be published on all aspects of clinical practice. In addition, from time to time when appropriate, these publications may be revised and updated. Thus, the series will provide quick access to relevant and important areas of psychiatric practice. Some books in the series will be authored by a person considered to be an expert in that particular area; others will be edited by such an expert, who will also draw together other knowledgeable authors to produce a comprehensive overview of that topic.

Some of the books in the Clinical Practice Series will have

their foundation in presentations at an annual meeting of the American Psychiatric Association. All will contain the most recently available information on the subjects discussed. Theoretical and scientific data will be applied to clinical situations, and case illustrations will be utilized in order to make the material even more relevant for the practitioner. Thus, the Clinical Practice Series should provide educational reading in a compact format especially designed for the mental health clinician-psychiatrist.

Judith H. Gold, M.D., F.R.C.P.C.
Series Editor

Clinical Practice Series Titles

Group Therapy for Schizophrenic Patients (#39)
By Nick Kanas, M.D.

Sexual Harassment in the Workplace and Academia: Psychiatric Issues (#38)
Edited by Diane K. Shrier, M.D.

Use of Neuroleptics in Children (#37)
Edited by Mary Ann Richardson, Ph.D., and Gary Haugland, M.A.

The New Pharmacotherapy of Schizophrenia (#36)
Edited by Alan Breier, M.D.

Clinical Assessment and Management of Severe Personality Disorders (#35)
Edited by Paul S. Links, M.D., M.Sc., F.R.C.P.C.

Predictors of Treatment Response in Mood Disorders (#34)
Edited by Paul J. Goodnick, M.D.

Successful Psychiatric Practice: Current Dilemmas, Choices, and Solutions (#33)
Edited by Edward K. Silberman, M.D.

Alternatives to the Hospital for Acute Psychiatric Treatment (#32)
Edited by Richard Warner, M.B., D.P.M.

Behavioral Complications in Alzheimer's Disease (#31)
Edited by Brian A. Lawlor, M.D.

Patient Violence and the Clinician (#30)
Edited by Burr S. Eichelman, M.D., Ph.D., and Anne C. Hartwig, J.D., Ph.D.

Effective Use of Group Therapy in Managed Care (#29)
Edited by K. Roy MacKenzie, M.D., F.R.C.P.C.

Rediscovering Childhood Trauma: Historical Casebook and Clinical Applications (#28)
Edited by Jean M. Goodwin, M.D., M.P.H.

Treatment of Adult Survivors of Incest (#27)
Edited by Patricia L. Paddison, M.D.

Madness and Loss of Motherhood: Sexuality, Reproduction, and Long-Term Mental Illness (#26)
Edited by Roberta J. Apfel, M.D., M.P.H., and Maryellen H. Handel, Ph.D.

Psychiatric Aspects of Symptom Management in Cancer Patients (#25)
Edited by William Breitbart, M.D., and Jimmie C. Holland, M.D.

Responding to Disaster: A Guide for Mental Health Professionals (#24)
Edited by Linda S. Austin, M.D.

Psychopharmacological Treatment Complications in the Elderly (#23)
Edited by Charles A. Shamoian, M.D., Ph.D.

Anxiety Disorders in Children and Adolescents (#22)
By Syed Arshad Husain, M.D., F.R.C.P.C., F.R.C.Psych., and Javad Kashani, M.D.

Suicide and Clinical Practice (#21)
Edited by Douglas Jacobs, M.D.

Special Problems in Managing Eating Disorders (#20)
Edited by Joel Yager, M.D., Harry E. Gwirtsman, M.D., and Carole K. Edelstein, M.D.

Children and AIDS (#19)
Edited by Margaret L. Stuber, M.D.

Current Treatments of Obsessive-Compulsive Disorder (#18)
Edited by Michele Tortora Pato, M.D., and Joseph Zohar, M.D.

Benzodiazepines in Clinical Practice: Risks and Benefits (#17)
Edited by Peter P. Roy-Byrne, M.D., and Deborah S. Cowley, M.D.

Adolescent Psychotherapy (#16)
Edited by Marcia Slomowitz, M.D.

Family Approaches in Treatment of Eating Disorders (#15)
Edited by D. Blake Woodside, M.D., M.Sc., F.R.C.P.C., and
Lorie Shekter-Wolfson, M.S.W., C.S.W.

Clinical Management of Gender Identity Disorders in Children and Adults (#14)
Edited by Ray Blanchard, Ph.D., and Betty W. Steiner, M.B., F.R.C.P.C.

New Perspectives on Narcissism (#13)
Edited by Eric M. Plakun, M.D.

The Psychosocial Impact of Job Loss (#12)
By Nick Kates, M.B.B.S., F.R.C.P.C., Barrie S. Greiff, M.D., and
Duane Q. Hagen, M.D.

Office Treatment of Schizophrenia (#11)
Edited by Mary V. Seeman, M.D., F.R.C.P.C., and
Stanley E. Greben, M.D., F.R.C.P.C.

Psychiatric Care of Migrants: A Clinical Guide (#10)
By Joseph Westermeyer, M.D., M.P.H., Ph.D.

Family Involvement in Treatment of the Frail Elderly (#9)
Edited by Marion Zucker Goldstein, M.D.

Measuring Mental Illness: Psychometric Assessment for Clinicians (#8)
Edited by Scott Wetzler, Ph.D.

Juvenile Homicide (#7)
Edited by Elissa P. Benedek, M.D., and Dewey G. Cornell, Ph.D.

The Neuroleptic Malignant Syndrome and Related Conditions (#6)
By Arthur Lazarus, M.D., Stephan C. Mann, M.D., and
Stanley N. Caroff, M.D.

Anxiety: New Findings for the Clinician (#5)
Edited by Peter Roy-Byrne, M.D.

Anxiety and Depressive Disorders in the Medical Patient (#4)
By Leonard R. Derogatis, Ph.D., and Thomas N. Wise, M.D.

Family Violence: Emerging Issues of a National Crisis (#3)
Edited by Leah J. Dickstein, M.D., and Carol C. Nadelson, M.D.

Divorce as a Developmental Process (#2)
Edited by Judith H. Gold, M.D., F.R.C.P.C.

Treating Chronically Mentally Ill Women (#1)
Edited by Leona L. Bachrach, Ph.D., and Carol C. Nadelson, M.D.

Introduction

Mary Ann Richardson, Ph.D.
Gary Haugland, M.A.

In this book on the use of neuroleptics in children, we have assembled reports from several professionals working in child psychiatry, pharmacology, and related fields; recent research they have been conducting; and new insights they have gained. The chapters deal with different aspects of the use of neuroleptics in this young population, from reviewing the existing literature to research spanning a statewide treatment system, from clinical trials of different medications to innovative laboratory approaches, interspersed with case studies revealing problematic issues.

In reading this entire book or the chapters of particular interest, the clinician should come away with greater knowledge of the role of neuroleptics and the potential problems, information that should be useful in making rational decisions regarding the prescribing of particular drugs. Often the chapters reveal that certain drugs are preferable to others, specific doses that have proved effective, titration schedules that are practical, and timely recognition of unwanted side effects.

The introduction of neuroleptics signaled a period of great progress in the reduction of the symptoms associated with severe psychiatric disorders. Although the greatest strides have been made in the amelioration of psychotic features of schizophrenia, many other illnesses have benefited from the actions of neuroleptics: the disruptive behaviors seen in conduct disorders and the uncontrolled outbursts of tics and repetitive stereotyped behaviors have all responded to neuroleptic treatment.

Campbell and Gonzalez's (Chapter 1) overview reveals that in the last four decades a tremendous amount of literature on the positive benefits of neuroleptics for children has been generated. In this book there are chapters on treatment issues related to Tourette's disorder (Shapiro and Shapiro, Chapter 7; Sallee, Rock, and Head, Chapter 8; Bruun and Budman, Chapter 9), autism (Malone, Chapter 6), schizophrenia (Spencer, Kafantaris, Padron-Gayol, and Rosenberg, Chapter 4), conduct disorder (Greenhill, Halperin, and Barmack, Chapter 5) as well as more general child psychiatric disorders (Zito, Craig, and Wanderling, Chapter 2; Richardson and Haugland, Chapter 3).

Perhaps no other children's disorder has benefited more from the introduction of neuroleptics than Tourette's disorder. With the virtual elimination of all but the most severe tics, children with this disorder have been able to function in classrooms and other public settings as never before. In autistic children, neuroleptics have reduced stereotypies and other behavioral symptoms and thus have facilitated learning, particularly the acquisition of language. The calming sedative effects of neuroleptics have controlled the disruptive behaviors of conduct disorders and the thought disorders of schizophrenia and allowed for increased attentiveness in the classroom.

These undeniable benefits of neuroleptic treatment, however, do have some undesirable side effects. Some of the most troublesome side effects—among them, oversedation, cognitive impairment, parkinsonism, emerging behavior problems—are examined in this book. Thus the benefits of the medication must always be tempered by the potential for adverse effects, and the clinician's task is to find the optimal balance of symptom reduction with a minimal of neuroleptic-induced side effects. This book offers the clinician guidelines for both the use of neuroleptics for particular children's disorders and how to recognize the undesired effects of the medication in this vulnerable population.

Diagnostic Issues

Which children are liable to receive neuroleptics? Neuroleptics are prescribed in children to address specific symptoms and not necessarily for particular syndromes or diagnostic entities. Some of the disorders described in this book follow the children into adulthood, sometimes becoming full-blown psychiatric diagnoses; others may fluctuate greatly over time and even completely remit.

It will become clear from these chapters that neuroleptics are prescribed for a great variety of reasons. The study by Spencer et al. (Chapter 4) is limited to children diagnosed with schizophrenia, arguably the most appropriate group to receive neuroleptics. As noted by Campbell and Gonzalez (Chapter 1), this is a very rare disorder in children and occurs only slightly more frequently among adolescents. In addition to schizophrenia, Zito et al. (Chapter 2) document the extent to which these medications are used for nonpsychotic disorders across a statewide inpatient population and that there may be gender differences as well. Campbell and Gonzalez's historic overview reveals that the literature has covered many diagnostic groups, but they are quick to point out that in children the key rationale for prescribing has been symptom-specific rather than disease-specific. Richardson and Haugland (Chapter 3) describe a cohort of children with a variety of psychiatric disorders. Greenhill et al. (Chapter 5) focus on nonpsychotic children with conduct disorders. This book will bring the clinician several steps closer to understanding the complexities of neuroleptic treatment in children and adolescents with different diagnoses.

Selecting Neuroleptics

The more concisely defined a particular disorder is, the more likely a narrow range of treatments will be promoted. The salient characteristics of Tourette's disorder are at present well known, and the quality of clinical research done has resulted in the role of neuroleptics being well understood. The work of Shapiro and Shapiro (Chapter 7) in particular has narrowed the specifications of those medications found to be most effective in reducing tics and other distressing manifestations of Tourette's disorder. The field is now addressing the unwanted side effects of these neuroleptics and, as Bruun and Budman (Chapter 9) and Sallee et al. (Chapter 8) both discuss, refining the dosing issues and the use of anticholinergic medications.

Sallee et al. (Chapter 8) describe a clinical trial comparing haloperidol and pimozide in the treatment of Tourette's; Malone (Chapter 6) describes these same two drugs for the treatment of autism. Such studies serve to identify particular neuroleptics with particular disorders and to understand the problems associated with any of the medications. As Sallee et al. point out, there seems to be a very narrow dose range between the therapeutic and the toxic.

Spencer et al. (Chapter 4) have been conducting an ongoing study of haloperidol administration in a young schizophrenic population. Although these children tend to retain their diagnoses over time, and thus the appropriateness of neuroleptic treatment cannot be challenged, nonetheless arriving at optimal doses requires constant vigilance on the part of the clinician. Zito et al. (Chapter 2) and Richardson and Haugland (Chapter 3) reveal the great diversity of disorders with which the clinician working in a public psychiatric hospital must contend. Thus it is ever more important that these psychiatrists be provided with the most up-to-date information to obtain the best possible care for these youngsters.

There are few generalizations that can be made; each child must be seen as an individual case. Even those with the same symptom clusters, or diagnoses, may have little in common, and their responses to medications, dosages, and changes in either are likely to be idiosyncratic. Campbell and Gonzalez (Chapter 1) recognize that clinicians often fall back on familiar drugs (often based on their experiences with adult patients) and may avoid the new and less familiar, such as lithium.

Untoward Side Effects

At the same time that the benefits of neuroleptics are being seen, a variety of side effects may emerge. One of these is of great concern to several authors contributing to this book on children—cognitive impairment. Although the sedating effects of neuroleptics can produce calm in previously disruptive children, the child's ability to remain attentive, absorb information, and solve problems may be compromised if the sedation is too great. Thus a significant body of work has been done to demonstrate which medications and at which doses minimize this problem while still attaining a desired level of symptom control. Greenhill et al. (Chapter 5) and Sallee et al. (Chapter 8) both address this concern and provide detailed reports on measuring cognitive functioning using the Continuous Performance Test. Although they express some reservations regarding the application of findings obtained in the laboratory to the complexities of classroom settings, they do offer hopeful approaches to deciding which neuroleptics may be optimally prescribed.

Another aspect of neuroleptic treatment that is addressed in this volume is behavioral change that may be a side effect of the medication. Bruun and Budman (Chapter 9) in particular show how patients with Tourette's disorder may over a period of time manifest outwardly distressing (and potentially dangerous) behaviors as a result of their neuroleptic treatment. Such changes are uncharacteristic enough that they leave the children themselves with the tough decision of whether to continue complying with their medication regimen for their tic disorders or to stop taking the neuroleptics and reverse their newly emerging behavior disorders. Clinicians can only hope to strike a balance that allows sufficient symptom reduction with a minimal impact on psychosocial functioning.

Tourette's disorder is dealt with in great detail by Shapiro and Shapiro (Chapter 7). In addition to presenting a broad overview of the disorder and its general treatment considerations, Shapiro and Shapiro describe the monitoring and management of adverse effects. Particular neuroleptics have come to the forefront in the treatment of Tourette's—haloperidol and pimozide, and to a lesser extent fluphenazine. Sallee et al. (Chapter 8) arrive at the conclusion that pimozide may be preferable despite the long history of successful treatment of Tourette's disorder with haloperidol.

The widespread underrecognition of Parkinson-like symptoms in patients with Tourette's disorder is mentioned by Bruun and Budman (Chapter 9), and the emergence of the movement disorders of tardive dyskinesia and parkinsonism in other psychiatric patients is described by Richardson and Haugland (Chapter 3). Atypicality in the emergence of side effects in patients treated with neuroleptics appears to be the norm. Thus clinicians must abandon many preconceived notions of the pharmacology of neuroleptic-induced movement disorders and expect the unexpected.

Monitoring and Assessing Patients

Several of the chapters address how medication effectiveness and the emergence of undesired side effects can be monitored during a course of treatment. Obviously a hospitalized population lends itself more readily to the kinds of techniques described. Nonetheless, it is critical that certain steps be taken to ensure that these effects be identified as soon as possible.

The importance of standard baseline measures prior to neuroleptic exposure was emphasized by several of the authors to identify changes due to the medication. School performance instruments have been used extensively in the assessment of cognitive functioning, but symptom checklists and behavior rating scales are also in evidence. As more investigators agree on which scales to use, the possibility of meaningful cross-study comparisons will become reality, and the field of child psychiatry will benefit greatly.

One key method that is gaining in prominence is the use of videotapes. Malone (Chapter 6) describes how baseline measures are augmented with a visual record of the patient's appearance obtained at the earliest possible time. Reliance on memory, even when complete clinical notes are available, may be less than ideal. With a videotape of a rating session, for example, changes over time can be detected much more readily, and even the most subtle side effects can be seen.

Computers also hold a significant place in the technology of child psychiatry. Computers are not just tools for the complex analysis of data, but they can serve as interactive techniques to test cognitive functioning in the realms of memory, attention, and eye-hand coordination. Both Greenhill et al. (Chapter 5) and Sallee et al. (Chapter 8) describe the Continuous Performance Test, a procedure that relies on the patient's direct interaction with computer images.

This book presents many stimulating chapters on issues surrounding the treatment of children and adolescents with neuroleptics. The heterogeneity of this patient population and the variety of responses, both good and bad, to medications serve to focus the psychiatrist on the importance of individualized treatment approaches to the use of neuroleptics in children.

CHAPTER 1

Overview of Neuroleptic Use in Child Psychiatric Disorders

Magda Campbell, M.D.
Nilda M. Gonzalez, M.D.

Unlike adult psychiatric patients, where the use of neuroleptics is restricted to schizophrenia and other psychotic conditions, children are receiving neuroleptics for a variety of psychiatric disorders. Since the advent of chlorpromazine 40 years ago (Delay and Deniker 1952), much knowledge has been gained about the efficacy and safety of neuroleptics in adult patients. These data are based on large and controlled clinical trials conducted in well-defined patient populations. Even though neuroleptics are widely used in children, with a few exceptions, systematic large-scale and long-term studies of neuroleptics are lacking in this age group of patients (for a comprehensive review, see Campbell et al. 1993).

After the introduction of chlorpromazine, reports on the use of neuroleptics in children were being seen in the literature by 1955. These reports were often uncontrolled studies with small patient samples involving children who were heterogeneous in terms of chronological age and diagnosis (Bair and Herold 1955; Freed and Peifer 1956; Freedman et al. 1955; Miksztal 1956; Rettig 1955). Instruments for emotionally disturbed children were not developed at the time, and the studies were poorly designed. Fish et al.'s (1966) study was a double-blind, controlled study of trifluoperazine involving 22 preschool-age autistic children. In this study a rating instrument was developed to test the relationship of initial severity of language impairment to neuroleptic treatment efficacy.

Valid and reliable assessment instruments have been developed for children and adolescents in the last two decades (see *Psychopharmacology Bulletin* 1973). These include the Conners Parent and Teacher Questionnaire and the Children's Psychiatric Rating Scale, both of which have been employed in double-blind, placebo-controlled clinical trials (L. T. Anderson et al. 1984, 1989; Campbell et al. 1978, 1984). Furthermore, the diagnostic criteria for psychiatric disorders in childhood were not spelled out until the development of DSM-III (American Psychiatric Association 1980). Still very much needed are studies on the determination of minimum effective doses and on the behavioral toxicity so often manifested in children before any neuroleptic-induced extrapyramidal/parkinsonian side effects appear, as well as systematic research on the effect of neuroleptics on cognition, learning, and academic performance.

Indications, Choice of Drug, and Dosage

In children, as in adult psychiatric patients, neuroleptics are indicated for Tourette's disorder (Shapiro et al. 1989), schizophrenia (Spencer et al. 1992) and other psychoses, and affective disorders (Geller et al. 1985). Psychoses are rarely seen in young children, but there is a marked increase in adolescence. In addition, neuroleptics are effective in a subgroup of children diagnosed as having autistic disorder with target symptoms of hyperactivity, aggressiveness, temper tantrums, irritability, stereotypies, and withdrawal (L. T. Anderson et al. 1984, 1989; Campbell et al. 1978; Perry et al. 1989b). Neuroleptics may also be therapeutically useful in nonpsychotic disorders, such as conduct disorder characterized by severe aggressiveness and explosiveness (Campbell et al. 1982, 1984), and in mentally retarded individuals with severely disruptive behaviors or with a concomitant psychiatric diagnosis such as schizophrenia (for review, see Campbell and Malone 1991). Although dextroamphetamine or methylphenidate is the drug of choice in attention-deficit/hyperactivity disorder, a neuroleptic may be indicated in those patients who fail to respond to stimulants or antidepressants. The superiority of haloperidol, thioridazine, and chlorpromazine over placebo in attention-deficit/hyperactivity disorder has been demonstrated in several studies (Gittelman-Klein et al. 1976; Rapoport et al. 1971; Werry et al. 1966, 1975).

In general, the high-potency drugs (e.g., haloperidol, pimozide) seem to be more desirable than the low-potency drugs (chlorpromazine, thioridazine). Chlorpromazine, for example, is contraindicated in children with seizure disorders; it has been found to increase the frequency of seizures in mentally retarded individuals with preexisting seizure disorder or to lower the seizure threshold (Tarjan et al. 1957). Thioridazine was reported to have decreased the frequency of seizures (Pregelj and Barkauskas 1967). There is some promising evidence in adult patients that pimozide is effective in reducing negative symptoms in schizophrenia (Baro and Dom 1976; Feinberg et al. 1988) and has a positive effect on learning or performance (Baro and Dom 1976). In a small sample of autistic children, pimozide was effective in decreasing behavioral symptoms in five autistic children with hypoactivity without sedative effect at therapeutic doses (Ernst et al. 1992).

Prior to placing a child or adolescent on a neuroleptic, baseline assessments should be conducted that include measurement of height and weight, basic laboratory screening, and evaluation of abnormal movements employing the Abnormal Involuntary Movements Scale (Kane et al. 1991). After a stable baseline, neuroleptic treatment should begin with a low starting dose, with small and gradual increments as shown in Table 1–1, to avoid an acute dystonic reaction and permit the full exploration of the therapeutic dose range of the drug. The *Physicians' Desk Reference* (Medical Economics 1992) should be used as a guideline for maximum dose; if side effects develop, the dose should be lowered, and the minimum therapeutically effective dose used. It is our recommendation that medication should be discontinued approximately every 6 months to determine whether further drug administration is required and to monitor the development of withdrawal dyskinesias, a neuroleptic-related side effect (Crane and Naranjo 1971; Gardos et al. 1978) usually reversible in children (Campbell et al. 1988).

Table 1–1. Suggested regulation of haloperidol dosage

Day	Time	Dose (mg)	Total daily dose (mg)
Monday	8 A.M.	0.25	0.25
Tuesday	8 A.M.	0.25	0.5
	4 P.M.	0.25	
Thursday	8 A.M.	0.5	0.5
Saturday	8 A.M.	0.5	0.75
	4 P.M.	0.25	
Monday	8 A.M.	0.5	1.0
	4 P.M.	0.5	
Wednesday	8 A.M.	0.75	1.25
	4 P.M.	0.5	
Friday	8 A.M.	0.75	1.5
	4 P.M.	0.75	
Monday	8 A.M.	1.0	1.75
	4 P.M.	0.75	
Wednesday	8 A.M.	1.0	2.0
	4 P.M.	1.0	
Friday	8 A.M.	1.25	2.25
	4 P.M.	1.0	
Monday	8 A.M.	1.25	2.5
	4 P.M.	1.25	
Wednesday	8 A.M.	1.5	2.75
	4 P.M.	1.25	
Friday	8 A.M.	1.5	3.0
	4 P.M.	1.5	

Table 1–2 gives an overview of the selected literature on the use of neuroleptics in children and adolescents. Of all neuroleptics, the most systematic studies of efficacy and safety have been done with haloperidol. At our present state of knowledge, haloperidol is most effective in acute schizophrenia, in Tourette's disorder, with a subgroup of autistic children, and with children having a conduct disorder with aggressiveness.

Schizophrenia

Schizophrenia is rare in children (J. C. Anderson et al. 1987; Burd and Kerbeshian 1987), and the true prevalence rate for this age group cannot be determined, although in adolescence there is a sharp increase in its incidence (Loranger 1984; for review, see Campbell et al. 1991). There have been a few open or retrospective studies of haloperidol in children and adolescents diagnosed as schizophrenic. Realmuto et al. (1984) reported that thiothixene is superior to thioridazine in chronic schizophrenic adolescents, although the effects were modest with both treatments. Siefen and Remschmidt's (1986) report is based on a chart review; it suggests that clozapine was effective in 21 patients with schizophrenia, 15 of whom had the paranoid type. Although the mean age of the sample was 18.1 years, 12 of the 21 patients were younger than age 18. There is one carefully designed, placebo-controlled, double-blind study in children younger than 12 years old (Spencer et al. 1992), and another in adolescents with acute schizophrenia or acute exacerbation of chronic schizophrenia (Pool et al. 1976). Certainly administration of haloperidol in conservative doses (0.02–0.12 mg/kg/day; chlorpromazine equivalent [CPZ-EQ] 1–6 mg/kg/day) is associated with reduction of several symptoms, including hallucinations and persecutory ideation (Spencer et al. 1992).

Bipolar Disorder and Psychotic Depression

Bipolar disorder is another psychiatric illness rarely seen in children younger than age 12, with an increase in adolescence (Loranger and Levine 1978). To the best of our knowledge, there are no reports on the use of neuroleptics in children with bipolar disorder. The only report on the use of neuroleptics in psychotic depression indicates that six delusionally depressed adolescents, ages 12–16 years, showed remission of delusional ideation within 2 weeks of chlorpromazine administration ranging from 50 to 100 mg/day (Geller et al. 1985).

Autistic Disorder

The superiority of haloperidol over placebo in autistic children ages 2–8 years was shown in 1978 by Campbell et al. and has since been replicated (L. T. Anderson et al. 1984, 1989; Cohen et al. 1980). Children with prominent symptoms of hyperactivity, aggressive-

Table 1–2. Overview of the representative literature

Neuroleptic	Authors	Age		Sample size	Diagnosis/ symptoms	Drug	Daily dose (mg)		Daily dose (mg/kg)	
		Range	Mean				Range	Mean	Range	Mean
Phenothiazines										
Piperidines	Pregelj and Barkauskas 1967	2–68	16.7–17.6	304 (68 with seizure disorders)	Mentally retarded with disruptive behavior	Thioridazine	10–800	150–200		
	Gittelman-Klein et al. 1976		8.55	155	Hyperactivity	Thioridazine	50–300	160	0.99–14.38	4.54
	Realmuto et al. 1984	11.75–18.75		21	Chronic schizophrenia	Thioridazine	91–228	178		3.3
Piperazines	Fish et al. 1966	2–6		22	Autism	Trifluoperazine	2–20			
	Faretra et al. 1970	5–12		60	Autism, psychosis	Fluphenazine	0.75–3.75			

	Engelhardt et al. 1973	6–12		30	Autism	Fluphenazine		10.4		
Aliphatics	Werry et al. 1966	7–13	8.5	39	Hyper-activity	Chlorprom-azine	150–200	106		
	Rapoport et al. 1971	4.5–10.5		19	Hyper-activity; aggres-siveness	Chlorprom-azine	75			
	Campbell et al. 1982	6–11.75	8.68	15	Hetero-geneous/ aggres-siveness & explo-siveness	Chlorprom-azine	100–200	150	2.8–5.79	
	Geller et al. 1985	12–17		6	Delusional depression	Chlorprom-azine	50–100			
Butyro-phenones	Spencer et al. 1992	5.5–11.75	8.89	14	Schizo-phrenia	Halo-peridol	0.5–3.5	1.77	0.02–0.12	0.058

(continued)

Table 1–2. Overview of the representative literature *(continued)*

Neuroleptic	Authors	Age		Sample size	Diagnosis/symptoms	Drug	Daily dose (mg)		Daily dose (mg/kg)	
		Range	Mean				Range	Mean	Range	Mean
	Pool et al. 1976	13–18	9.8	75	Acute schizophrenia or exacerbation	Haloperidol	4.0–16.0	9.8		
	Cunningham et al. 1968	7.8–12.10		12	Conduct disorder	Haloperidol	0.5–3.0			
	Campbell et al. 1984	5.2–12.9	8.97	61	Conduct disorder	Haloperidol	1.0–6.0	2.95		
	Wong and Cock 1971	7–12		28	Conduct disorder	Haloperidol	0.05			
	Werry et al. 1975	4.92–12.33	7.75	29	ADHD/conduct disorder	Haloperidol	0.025	0.05		

	Campbell et al. 1978	2.6–7.2	4.5	40	Autism	Halo-peridol	0.5–4.0	1.65		
	L. T. Anderson et al. 1984	2.33–6.92	4.58	40	Autism	Halo-peridol	0.5–3.0	1.11	0.019–0.217	0.05
	L. T. Anderson et al. 1989	2.02–7.58	4.49	45	Autism	Halo-peridol	0.25–4.0	0.844	0.016–0.184	0.047
	Naruse et al. 1982	3–16		87	Hetero-geneous (34 with autism)	Halo-peridol	0.75–3.0			
	Perry et al. 1989a	2.3–7.9	5.1	82	Autism	Halo-peridol	0.5–4.0	1.23	0.016–0.209	0.059
	Shapiro et al. 1989	8–65	21.1 ± 11.0	57	Tourette's disorder	Halo-peridol	?–10	4.5 ± 2.7	?–0.17	0.08 ± 0.05
Thioxan-thenes	Campbell et al. 1970	3–7		10	Autism	Thio-thixene	1.0–6.0	2.0		

(continued)

Table 1–2. Overview of the representative literature *(continued)*

Neuroleptic	Authors	Age		Sample size	Diagnosis/symptoms	Drug	Daily dose (mg)		Daily dose (mg/kg)	
		Range	Mean				Range	Mean	Range	Mean
	Realmuto et al. 1984	11.75–18.75		21	Chronic schizophrenia	Thiothixene	4.8–42.6	16.2		0.3
Dihydroindolones	Campbell et al. 1971	3–5		10	Autism	Molindone	1.0–2.5			1.5
	Greenhill et al. 1985	6–11	9.8–10.3	31	Undersocialized conduct disorder, aggressive type	Molindone	25–?	26.8	0.5–2.0	1.3
Dibenzoxazepines	Pool et al. 1976	13–18		75	Acute schizophrenia or exacerbation	Loxapine	25–200	87.5		

Diphenylbutylpiperidine	Naruse et al. 1982	3–16		87	Heterogeneous (34 with autism)	Pimozide	1.0–5.0 for ages 3–5; 1.0–6.0 for ages 6–11; 1.0–9.0 for ages 12–16			
	Ernst et al. 1992	4.17–8.25	5.72	8	Autism	Pimozide	3.0–6.0	4.88	0.12–0.32	0.22
	Shapiro et al. 1989	8–65	21.1 ± 11.0	57	Tourette's disorder	Pimozide	?–20	10.6 ± 7.1	0.02–0.51	0.18 ± 0.12
	White and Aman 1985		15.7	8	Mental retardation with disruptive behaviors	Pimozide	6.0	0.12	0.09–0.18	
Dibenzodiazepine	Siefen and Remschmidt 1986		18.1	21	Schizophrenia, paranoid type	Clozapine	254–700	352		

Note. ADHD = attention-deficit/hyperactivity disorder.

ness, temper tantrums, irritability, self-injurious behavior, stereotypies, and social withdrawal seem to be the best responders (see also Locascio et al. 1991; Perry et al. 1989b). In no study was reduction of behavioral symptoms of haloperidol accompanied by adverse cognitive effects on performance or learning. Quite to the contrary, discrimination learning was facilitated by haloperidol (L. T. Anderson et al. 1984), and acquisition of words was increased when used in conjunction with language therapy (Campbell et al. 1978). Haloperidol remains effective in reducing symptoms when administered on a long-term basis (Perry et al. 1989b), and increases of IQ scores have been reported (Die Trill et al. 1984). However, clinical experience has shown that in those children who are not hyperactive, administration of haloperidol was associated with sedation in the absence of symptom reduction. In such children, pimozide seems to be a promising agent (Ernst et al. 1992), and it appears to be less sedative than haloperidol (Ernst et al. 1992; Freeman 1979; Ross and Moldofsky 1978). Furthermore, in children with Tourette's disorder, as well as in adults with chronic schizophrenia (Baro and Dom 1976), pimozide has shown beneficial effects on performance and learning.

The limitation of haloperidol is its association with tardive and withdrawal dyskinesia in about 12%–29% of children (Campbell et al. 1983, 1988, 1990; Malone et al. 1991; Meiselas et al. 1989; Perry et al. 1989a, 1989b; Richardson et al. 1991). These movement disorders appear most often after drug withdrawal and as early as after 56 days of cumulative exposure to haloperidol, although there are reports of patients who had been receiving haloperidol cumulatively for 7 years without showing dyskinetic movements (Campbell et al. 1988). Neuroleptics other than haloperidol, including pimozide, have also been associated with dyskinesia (Falloon et al. 1978).

Conduct Disorder, Aggressive type

Although there is some supportive evidence that lithium is superior to placebo in reducing aggressiveness, temper outbursts, and explosiveness in children diagnosed with conduct disorder and that lithium is favored over haloperidol because it lacks sedative effects at therapeutic doses (Campbell et al. 1984), some clinicians may prefer to use haloperidol or chlorpromazine because they are more familiar with this type of drug. Both chlorpromazine (Campbell et al. 1982) and haloperidol (Campbell et al. 1982, 1984) were found to be therapeutically effective in a population of children, although sedation at therapeutic doses may limit their usefulness. Effects of haloperidol on cognition and performance in the laboratory appear to depend on the dose employed: at lower doses, performance is facilitated (Werry and Aman 1975), whereas higher doses produce mildly negative effects (Platt et al. 1984; Werry and Aman 1975). Molindone also appears to be a promising agent in the treatment of children with conduct disorders, as reported by Greenhill et al. (1985).

Mental Retardation With Disruptive Behavior or Associated With Psychiatric Disorder (Dual Diagnosis)

Neuroleptics are widely used in developmentally disordered patient populations, whether institutionalized or living in the community (Intagliata and Rimck 1985). However, this is an understudied population, and only in recent years has there been a concern whether long-term neuroleptic treatment is justified in this population before efficacy and safety issues have been determined through rigorous research methods (see Aman and Singh 1991; Campbell and Malone 1991).

In persons of subnormal intellectual functioning, the effect of neuroleptics on cognition is of particular concern (Aman 1984). In general, the effectiveness of neuroleptics in reducing maladaptive behaviors is modest, and there seems to be little or no therapeutic advantage in giving higher rather than lower doses of haloperidol (Aman et al. 1989) or thioridazine (Singh and Aman 1981).

Tourette's Disorder

Although the superiority of haloperidol and of pimozide has been demonstrated for children with Tourette's disorder (Shapiro et al. 1989), the use of neuroleptics in these patients is limited by excessive sedation, possible adverse effects on cognition (Borison et al. 1982), and behavioral toxicity (Bruun 1988). By lowering the dose, their effectiveness in reducing the vocal and motor tics is reduced too (A. Shapiro, personal communication, May 1976).

Special Considerations in Outpatient Treatment

Although it is preferable from the clinical perspective to treat patients in an inpatient setting, which provides maximum control over the administration and monitoring of medication, this is not always possible or desirable. Increasingly, outpatient treatment for all but the most acute manifestations of a psychiatric illness is being recommended. There are, however, significant confounding problems in the outpatient treatment of children and adolescents that need to be discussed—in particular, monitoring of medication effects and assuring compliance with the prescribed drug regimen.

Monitoring

The most frequent problem with the use of neuroleptics in the practice of child psychiatry is overmedication, and this may be especially true in outpatient treatment environments, where the clinician cannot be expected to monitor the patient on a daily basis. When a patient is beginning a course of treatment with neuroleptics, it is critical to monitor the patient for desired and undesired effects of the drug. In the early stages of drug treatment, small, possibly subtherapeutic doses, are administered, and the dosage is increased slowly. Initially these are administered several times daily to allow for titration in small increments until a single therapeutically effective dose can be determined and to allow for early detection of side effects.

At baseline and throughout the course of treatment, clinical observation and quantitative assessment are an integral part of the treatment. During the dosage regulation period, before an optimal level has been determined, it is crucial to be aware of behavioral toxicity, which can appear before desired effects or other side effects emerge (Campbell and Deutsch 1985; Campbell et al. 1993). This may be manifest as an increase in problematic behaviors, even of those behaviors being treated with the neuroleptic in the first place.

When the patient is being treated in an institutional setting, it is clear that the staff can monitor this process frequently. If the patient is being treated as an outpatient, this requires the close cooperation of parents and teachers with the clinician to maintain daily observations of the patient (Campbell and Deutsch 1985). There are several scales that can be used by parents and teachers to record their impressions and when used consistently can reflect both the effectiveness of the medication in reducing problematic behaviors and the presence of any cognitive or behavioral side effects (for an inventory of such scales, see Campbell and Deutsch 1985). Furthermore, although the observations of parents and teachers are important, the ongoing subjective feelings of the child or adolescent patient must also be elicited.

Compliance

As soon as an effective dose level has been determined, it should be prescribed in a single daily dose to facilitate compliance and spare any possible embarrassment resulting from having to take medications during school hours. A single evening dose before sleep is not recommended, however. With a single bedtime dosage schedule, behavioral and other effects occurring at peak blood levels may be missed, and the risk of failing to recognize a serious acute dystonic reaction is increased (Campbell et al. 1985).

There are many reasons for noncompliance with medication regimens in psychiatric patients, and it is obviously easier to avoid taking medications as an outpatient. Although there may be unwanted side effects, these are primarily discomforting but not life threatening. This discomfort may be exacerbated in young patients, who are extremely sensitive to changes in their bodies and the reactions of their peers. Thus when the effects of the neuroleptics are perceived to interfere with normal social development and peer acceptance, the child or adolescent may choose to sacrifice the benefits of the medication. Side effects such as sedation, rigidity, or restlessness may be doubly distressing for young patients who have to be concerned with the impressions of others as well as their own subjective states.

In adult outpatients, depot preparations are frequently prescribed in cases where compliance is an issue. However, these are not recommended for use in children and adolescents because there is a lack of knowledge about their efficacy and safety in this population (Campbell et al. 1993).

Once medication use has been established, it is possible to

detect noncompliance through an awareness of medication withdrawal symptoms, including anorexia, nausea, vomiting, diarrhea, weight loss, and diaphoresis (Campbell et al. 1993). It is important again that the parents of the child or adolescent be able to report these to the clinician as part of the ongoing monitoring of the medication effects and as a way of ascertaining compliance. The most important deterrent to noncompliance is for the patient to have an understanding and acceptance of the intended effects of the medication and to recognize that the side effects, although unpleasant, are most likely only temporary.

Conclusion

Considering the wide use of neuroleptics in children and adolescents, further research in this area is warranted. Neurotransmitter abnormalities underlying various disorders should continue to be studied so that selection of potentially effective drugs can be based on a rational pharmacological basis (Deutsch and Campbell 1986). The relationship between plasma levels of neuroleptics and clinical response should be investigated to provide additional laboratory tests for monitoring. The effect of dosage on both symptom reduction and developmental features such as cognition must be considered, particularly when long-term drug maintenance is indicated. Above all, studies are required that compare pharmacological and psychosocial treatments and the interactive effect of the two approaches.

Neuroleptic-related dyskinesias represent the most serious drawback. However, the immediate benefits may outweigh the perceived untoward effects, especially because it is known that these effects are most often reversible. In young autistic children with target symptoms of aggressiveness and hyperactivity, haloperidol remained effective when administered on a long-term basis without negative effects on IQ (Gonzalez et al. 1992). Some of these children were mainstreamed without further medication, and the drug-related dyskinesias were found to be reversible over time. When long-term administration of a neuroleptic is warranted, a baseline screening for abnormal movements is required (Campbell 1985; Campbell and Palij 1985) and the long-term extrapyramidal side effects must be monitored regularly. When prescribed judiciously and monitored carefully, neuroleptics can play an important role in the comprehensive treatment program of the moderately to severely disturbed child, particularly when used in conjunction with special education programs, psychosocial treatment, and ongoing work with the family.

References

Aman MG: Drugs and learning in mentally retarded persons, in Advances in Human Psychopharmacology, Vol 3. Edited by Burrows GD, Werry JS. Greenwich CT, JAI Press, 1984, pp 121–163

Aman MG, Singh NN: Pharmacological intervention, in Handbook of Mental Retardation, 2nd Edition. Edited by Matson JL, Mulick JA. Elmsford, NY, Pergamon, 1991, pp 347–372

Aman MG, Teehan CJ, White AJ, et al: Haloperidol treatment with chronically medicated residents: dose effects on clinical behavior and reinforcement contingencies. Am J Ment Retard 95:452–460, 1989

American Psychiatric Association: Diagnostic and Statistical Manual of Mental Disorders, 3rd Edition. Washington, DC, American Psychiatric Association, 1980

Anderson JC, Williams S, McGee R, et al: DSM-III disorders in preadolescent children. Arch Gen Psychiatry 44:69–76, 1987

Anderson LT, Campbell M, Grega DM, et al: Haloperidol in the treatment of infantile autism: effects on learning and behavioral symptoms. Am J Psychiatry 141:1195–1202, 1984

Anderson LT, Campbell M, Adams P, et al: The effects of haloperidol on discrimination learning and behavioral symptoms in autistic children. J Autism Dev Disord 19:227–239, 1989

Bair HV, Herold W: Efficacy of chlorpromazine in hyperactive mentally retarded children. Archives of Neurology and Psychiatry 74:363–364, 1955

Baro F, Dom R: The interaction between neuroleptic treatment and sociotherapeutic approach in chronic schizophrenics: investigations with haloperidol, penfluridol and pimozide. Acta Psychiatr Belg 76:735–758, 1976

Borison RL, Ang L, Chang S, et al: New pharmacological approaches in the treatment of Tourette syndrome, in Gilles de la Tourette Syndrome: Advances in Neurology. Edited by Friedhoff W, Chase TN. New York, Raven, 1982, pp 377–382

Bruun RD: Subtle and underrecognized side effects of neuroleptic treatment in children with Tourette's Disorder. Am J Psychiatry 145:621–624, 1988

Burd L, Kerbeshian J: A North Dakota prevalence study of schizophrenia presenting in childhood. J Am Acad Child Adolesc Psychiatry 26:347–350, 1987

Campbell M: Protocol for rating drug-related AIMS, stereotypies and CPRS assessments (special feature). Psychopharmacol Bull 21:1081, 1985

Campbell M, Deutsch SI: Neuroleptics in children, in Drugs in Psychiatry, Vol 3: Antipsychotics. Edited by Burrows GD, Norman T, Davies B. Amsterdam, Elsevier Biomedical Press, 1985, pp 213–238

Campbell M, Malone RP: Mental retardation and psychiatric disorders. Hosp Community Psychiatry 42:374–379, 1991

Campbell M, Palij M: Measurement of untoward effects including tardive dyskinesia. Psychopharmacol Bull 21:1063–1082, 1985

Campbell M, Fish B, Shapiro T, et al: Thiothixene in young disturbed children: a pilot study. Arch Gen Psychiatry 23:70–72, 1970

Campbell M, Fish B, Shapiro T, et al: Study of molindone in disturbed preschool children. Current Therapeutic Research 13:28–33, 1971

Campbell M, Anderson LT, Meier M, et al: A comparison of haloperidol, behavior therapy and their interaction in autistic children. Journal of the American Academy of Child Psychiatry 17:640–655, 1978

Campbell M, Cohen IL, Small AM: Drugs in aggressive behavior. Journal of the American Academy of Child Psychiatry 21:107–117, 1982

Campbell M, Grega DM, Green WH, et al: Neuroleptic-induced dyskinesias in children. Clin Neuropharmacol 6:207–222, 1983

Campbell M, Small AM, Green WH, et al: Behavioral efficacy of haloperidol and lithium carbonate: a comparison in hospitalized aggressive children with conduct disorder. Arch Gen Psychiatry 41:650–656, 1984

Campbell M, Green WH, Deutsch SI (eds): Child and Adolescent Psychopharmacology. Beverly Hills, CA, Sage, 1985

Campbell M, Adams P, Perry R, et al: Tardive and withdrawal dyskinesia in autistic children: a prospective study. Psychopharmacol Bull 24:251–255, 1988

Campbell M, Locascio JJ, Choroco MC, et al: Stereotypies and tardive dyskinesia: abnormal movements in autistic children. Psychopharmacol Bull 26:260–266, 1990

Campbell M, Spencer EK, Kowalik SC, et al: Schizophrenic and psychotic disorders, in Textbook of Child and Adolescent Psychiatry. Edited by Wiener JM. Washington, DC, American Psychiatric Press, 1991, pp 223–239

Campbell M, Gonzalez NM, Ernst M, et al: Antipsychotics, in Practitioner's Guide to Psychoactive Drugs in Children and Adolescents. Edited by Werry JS, Aman M. New York, Plenum, 1993, pp 269–296

Cohen IL, Campbell M, Posner D, et al: Behavioral effects of haloperidol in young autistic children: an objective analysis using a within-subjects reversal design. Journal of the American Academy of Child Psychiatry 19:665–677, 1980

Crane GE, Naranjo ER: Motor disorders induced by neuroleptics. Arch Gen Psychiatry 24:178–184, 1971

Cunningham MA, Pillai V, Rogers WJB: Haloperidol in the treatment of children with severe behavioural disorders. Br J Psychiatry 114:845–854, 1968

Delay J, Deniker P: 38 cas de psychoses traitees par la cure prolongee et continue de 4560 RP-CR. 50ieme Congres des Alien et Neurologique de Langue Francaise, Luxembourg, 21–27 Juillet, 1952, p 503

Deutsch SI, Campbell M: Relative affinities for different classes of neurotransmitter receptors predict neuroleptic efficacy in infantile autism: a hypothesis. Neuropsychobiology 15:160–164, 1986

Die Trill ML, Wolsky BB, Shell J, et al: Effects of long term haloperidol treatment on intellectual functioning in autistic children: a pilot study. Paper presented at the 31st Annual Meeting of the American Academy of Child Psychiatry, Toronto, Canada, October 10–14, 1984

Engelhardt DM, Polizos P, Waizer J, et al: A double-blind comparison of fluphenazine and haloperidol in outpatient schizophrenic children. Journal of Autism and Childhood Schizophrenia 3:128–137, 1973

Ernst M, Magee HJ, Gonzalez NM, et al: Pimozide in autistic children. Psychopharmacol Bull 28:187–191, 1992

Falloon I, Watt DC, Shepherd M: A comparative controlled trial of pimozide and fluphenazine decanoate in the continuation therapy of schizophrenia. Psychol Med 8:59–70, 1978

Faretra G, Dooher L, Dowling J: Comparison of haloperidol and fluphenazine in disturbed children. Am J Psychiatry 126:1670–1673, 1970

Feinberg SS, Kay SR, Elijovich LR, et al: Pimozide treatment of the negative schizophrenic syndrome: an open trial. J Clin Psychiatry 49:235–238, 1988

Fish B, Shapiro T, Campbell M: Long-term prognosis and the response of schizophrenic children to drug therapy: a controlled study of trifluoperazine. Am J Psychiatry 123:32–39, 1966

Freed H, Peifer CA: Treatment of hyperkinetic emotionally disturbed children with prolonged administration of chlorpromazine. Am J Psychiatry 113:22–26, 1956

Freedman AM, Effron AS, Bender L: Pharmacotherapy in children with psychiatric illness. J Nerv Ment Dis 122:479–486, 1955

Freeman H: Pimozide as a neuroleptic. Br J Psychiatry 135:82–83, 1979

Gardos G, Cole J, Tarsy D: Withdrawal symptoms associated with antipsychotic drugs. Am J Psychiatry 135:1321–1324, 1978

Geller B, Cooper TB, Farooki ZQ, et al: Dose and plasma levels of nortriptyline and chlorpromazine in delusionally depressed adolescents and of nortriptyline in nondelusionally depressed adolescents. Am J Psychiatry 142:336–338, 1985

Gittelman-Klein R, Klein DF, Katz S, et al: Comparative effects of methylphenidate and thioridazine in hyperkinetic children, I: clinical results. Arch Gen Psychiatry 33:1217–1231, 1976

Gonzalez NM, Alpert M, Shay J, et al: DSM-IV Field Trial: change of diagnosis in autistic children on follow-up. Paper presented at the annual meeting of the American College of Neuropsychopharmacology, San Juan, Puerto Rico, December 1992

Greenhill LL, Solomon M, Pleak R, et al: Molindone hydrochloride treatment of hospitalized children with conduct disorder. J Clin Psychiatry 46:20–25, 1985

Intagliata J, Rimck C: Psychoactive drug use in public and community residential facilities for mentally retarded persons. Psychopharmacol Bull 21:268–278, 1985

Kane J, Jeste DU, Barnes TRE, et al: Tardive Dyskinesia: A Task Force Report of the American Psychiatric Association. Washington, DC, American Psychiatric Association, 1991

Locascio JJ, Malone RP, Small AS, et al: Factors related to haloperidol response and dyskinesias in autistic children. Psychopharmacol Bull 27:119–126, 1991

Loranger AW: Sex difference in age at onset of schizophrenia. Arch Gen Psychiatry 41:157–161, 1984

Loranger AW, Levine PM: Age at onset of bipolar affective illness. Arch Gen Psychiatry 35:1345–1348, 1978

Malone RP, Ernst M, Godfrey KA, et al: Repeated episodes of neuroleptic-related dyskinesias in autistic children. Psychopharmacol Bull 27:113–117, 1991

Medical Economics Co: Physicians' Desk Reference, 46th Edition. Oradell, NJ, Medical Economics, 1992

Meiselas KD, Spencer EK, Oberfield R, et al: Differentiation of stereotypies from neuroleptic-related dyskinesias in autistic children. J Clin Psychopharmacol 9:207–209, 1989

Miksztal MW: Chlorpromazine (Thorazine) and reserpine in residential treatment of neuropsychiatric disorders in children. J Nerv Ment Dis 123:477–479, 1956

Naruse H, Nagahata M, Nakane Y, et al: A multicenter double-blind trial of pimozide (Orap), haloperidol and placebo in children with behavioral disorders, using crossover design. Acta Paedopsychiatrica 48:173–184, 1982

Perry R, Nobler MS, Campbell M: Case report: Tourette-like symptoms associated with chronic neuroleptic therapy in an autistic child. J Am Acad Child Adolesc Psychiatry 28:93–96, 1989a

Perry R, Campbell M, Adams P, et al: Long-term efficacy of haloperidol in autistic children: continuous versus discontinuous drug administration. J Am Acad Child Adolesc Psychiatry 28:87–92, 1989b

Platt JE, Campbell M, Green WH, et al: Cognitive effects of lithium carbonate and haloperidol in treatment-resistant aggressive children. Arch Gen Psychiatry 41:657–662, 1984

Pool D, Bloom W, Mielke DH, et al: A controlled evaluation of Loxitane in seventy-five adolescent schizophrenic patients. Current Therapeutic Research 19:99–104, 1976

Pregelj S, Barkauskas A: Thioridazine in the treatment of mentally retarded children: a four-year retroactive evaluation. Journal of the Canadian Psychiatric Association 12:213–215, 1967

Psychopharmacology Bulletin: Pharmacotherapy of Children (Special Issue). Psychopharmacol Bull 9:1–241, 1973

Rapoport J, Abramson A, Alexander D, et al: Playroom observations of hyperactive children on medication. Journal of the American Academy of Child Psychiatry 10:524–534, 1971

Realmuto GM, Erickson WD, Yellin A, et al: Clinical comparison of thiothixene and thioridazine in schizophrenic adolescents. Am J Psychiatry 141:440–442, 1984

Rettig JH: Chlorpromazine for the control of psychomotor excitement in the mentally deficient: a preliminary study. J Nerv Ment Dis 122:190–194, 1955

Richardson MA, Haugland G, Craig TJ: Neuroleptic use, parkinsonian symptoms, tardive dyskinesia, and associated factors in child and adolescent psychiatric patients. Am J Psychiatry 148:1322–1328, 1991

Ross MS, Moldofsky H: A comparison of pimozide and haloperidol in the treatment of Gilles de la Tourette's syndrome. Am J Psychiatry 135:585–587, 1978

Shapiro E, Shapiro AK, Fulop G, et al: Controlled study of haloperidol, pimozide, and placebo for the treatment of Gilles de la Tourette's syndrome. Arch Gen Psychiatry 46:722–730, 1989

Siefen G, Remschmidt H: Behandllungsergebnisse mit clozapin bei schizophrenen Jugendlichen. Z Kinder Jugendpsychiatr 14:245–257, 1986

Singh NN, Aman MG: Effects of thioridazine dosage on the behavior of severely mentally retarded persons. American Journal of Mental Deficiency 85:580–587, 1981

Spencer EK, Kafantaris V, Padron-Gayol M, et al: Haloperidol in schizophrenic children: early findings from a study in progress. Psychopharmacol Bull 28:183–186, 1992

Tarjan C, Lowery VE, Wright SW: Use of chlorpromazine in two hundred seventy-eight mentally deficient patients. American Medical Association Journal of Disturbed Children 94:294–300, 1957

Werry JS, Aman MG: Methylphenidate and haloperidol in children: effects on attention, memory and activity. Arch Gen Psychiatry 32:790–795, 1975

Werry JS, Weiss G, Douglas V, et al: Studies on the hyperactive child, III: the effect of chlorpromazine upon behavior and learning ability. Journal of the American Academy of Child Psychiatry 5:292–312, 1966

Werry JS, Aman MG, Lampen E: Haloperidol and methylphenidate in hyperactive children. Acta Paedopsychiatrica 42:26–40, 1975

White AJ, Aman MG: Pimozide treatment in disruptive severely retarded patients. Aust N Z J Psychiatry 19:92–94, 1985

Wong GH, Cock RJ: Long-term effects of haloperidol on severely emotionally disturbed children. Aust N Z J Psychiatry 5:296–300, 1971

CHAPTER 2

Neuroleptic Use in Children and Adolescents Hospitalized for Psychiatric Disorders: Gender Issues and Implications

Julie Magno Zito, Ph.D.
Thomas J. Craig, M.D., M.P.H.
Joseph A. Wanderling, M.A.

Neuroleptic use in children and adolescents has been the subject of much scrutiny as our knowledge of neuroleptic benefits and risks has grown. Despite this general interest, research has been limited. A brief review of the pediatric psychopharmacological literature (Biederman 1992; Campbell et al. 1985; Green 1991) reveals a general consensus that, compared with adults, children and adolescents are the subject of fewer empirical psychopharmacological studies and that clinical trials are particularly lacking. For example, there have been no studies of the efficacy of neuroleptics in childhood schizophrenia (American Psychiatric Association 1992), and clinical experience has reported less benefit in children than in adolescents or adults with schizophrenia (Campbell and Spencer 1988). This more scant experience has led to a weaker knowledge base from which psychopharmacological practice standards are derived. The relative lack of research information on dosage guidelines may lead to extrapolation from adult findings (Simeon 1989) despite the potential for differences in developmental disposition (Jatlow 1987), including pharmacokinetics and pharmacodynamic factors that might alter the drug's effect in children (Teicher and Baldessarini 1987).

In the absence of clinical trials to gain more knowledge of the prescribing and dosing patterns in children and adolescents, naturalistic studies provide one of the only sources of information on the effects and effectiveness of psychotropic agents in these age groups. The paucity of epidemiological data on psychotropic prescribing in this age group has been noted (Waters 1990). A recent review of the clinical literature produced few surveys of pediatric psychopharmacology, most of which were conducted outside the United States and focused on specific questions among outpatients. For example, reports have examined the prescribing practices of primary care physicians compared with child psychiatry consultants (Adams 1991) or the prevalence of psychotropic drugs in outpatients (Elliger et al. 1990; Quinn 1986). The utility of these studies is further limited by the outpatient population and the lack of diagnostic information provided.

To address the issue of the prevalence of psychotropic prescriptions among more seriously ill young people, we conducted a study of children and adolescents hospitalized at four public psychiatric facilities for major mental disorders during a 3-month period (Zito et al. 1994). Some form of medication, whether scheduled or on an as-needed (prn) basis, was prescribed for 98% of a cohort initially consisting of 501 patients. All patients meeting length of hospitalization and diagnostic criteria who received scheduled psychotropic medication ($N = 267$) were evaluated regarding two hypotheses: 1) that children and adolescent patients, similar to adult inpatients, will experience drug regimens that become more complex as their time in hospital increases and 2) that hospitalized children and adolescents, also like adult patients, will receive higher doses of neuroleptics as their time in hospital increases. Both hypotheses were supported by the study findings, replicating our previous adult findings (Zito et al. 1988) and supporting a model for neuroleptic drug prescription in which diagnosis, potency group, and length of hospitalization are key factors.

More specifically, the study findings in children and adolescents showed significantly greater neuroleptic ($P < .0001$) and anticholinergic ($P < .05$) exposure among schizophrenic short-stay patients compared with other short-stay diagnostic groups. In addition, neuroleptic usage was considerably greater ($P < .0001$) among long-stay patients with conduct (74% versus 20%), affective (73% versus 18%), and adjustment/personality (92% versus 9%) disorders when compared with their short-stay counterparts. Finally, there was no significant difference in prevalence of neuroleptic use among the long-stay patients according to diagnosis. These findings of relatively widespread use of neuroleptics regardless of diagnosis among long-stay patients were not anticipated and suggest a need for more controlled studies of the effectiveness of psychotropics for unlabeled indications (Collins et al. 1991).

The role of gender in psychopharmacological drug evaluation has not been given much attention until recently (Yonkers et al. 1992). These authors concluded that gender differences in regard to the prescription of psychotherapeutic agents is a topic occasionally, but incompletely, addressed by past studies. Early community surveys (Cooperstock 1971; Craig and Van Natta 1978; Parry et al. 1973) supported the greater prescription of psychotherapeutic agents for women compared with men. When the type of psychotropic was considered, preferential prescribing for women was seen for minor tranquilizers but was not observed for neuroleptics and antidepressants (Parry et al. 1973). A decade later, this finding was replicated (Hohmann 1989) in an analysis that ruled out statistically significant differences in presenting symptoms, physicians' diagnoses, and sociodemographic and health service factors as possible explanations of the differential effect in prescribing for women.

Although it is generally believed that gender bias does not occur in regard to the selection of neuroleptics, whether it influences neuroleptic dosage is controversial. Previous studies show conflicting findings of decreased dosage (Young and Meltzer 1980), increased dosage (Zito et al. 1987), and no difference (Seeman 1986) in dosing by gender. In the latter case, no difference in dosage was observed for premenopausal women compared with young men, whereas older women received *greater* doses than age-matched men. Several small studies have reported higher plasma levels for women on a given neuroleptic dose (Ereshefsky et al. 1991; Simpson et al. 1990) or on lower doses (Chouinard et al. 1986), but they failed to control for concurrent medication usage, making inferences about the neuroleptic and its effectiveness uninterpretable.

Studies conducted among adults have led some researchers to suggest an underlying biological basis for the observed differential usage. For example, the antidopaminergic effect of estrogen was postulated (Seeman 1986) to explain the lower doses seen among young women compared with older women. Unfortunately, there are many competing clinical factors (e.g., length of neuroleptic exposure, drug tolerance, severity of illness) that may explain the dose differential. In addition, physicians' attitudes and prescribing practice differences (Lehmann 1968) and bias in regard to gender-related behaviors (e.g., perceived need for larger doses in males to control aggression) may further erode a biological model for the observed gender differences in dosing.

The children's psychopharmacological literature has not addressed the gender issue, in part because the study populations in clinical trials predominantly have been male in composition and the study samples have been small (M. Campbell, personal communication, December 1990). It is not until adulthood that prevalence of mental disorders becomes more balanced in regard to gender. Because it is unlikely that prospective studies will be carried out to address questions of gender bias, the present study of neuroleptic usage in youngsters hospitalized for severe mental disorders utilized the data set described above to address gender bias. Following the hypothesis generated by adult gender bias studies, this study considers whether young females received fewer psychotropic agents than males after accounting for differences in diagnosis. Second, the data are examined for differences in neuroleptic dosing between the genders after accounting for the influence of age and diagnosis. The discussion also reviews gender-related findings in the context of previous data regarding neuroleptic usage and length of hospitalization.

Method

The study group was selected from a total cohort of 501 individual patients in the hospital during a 3-month interval (January 1 through March 31, 1990) in four child/adolescent inpatient treatment settings operated by the New York State Office of Mental Health. Data from a computerized information system were used to characterize each patient in the study group according to gender, age, diagnosis, class of psychotropic medication ordered, daily dose of neuroleptic administered, and length of the current hospitalization. The most recent DSM-III-R (American Psychiatric Association 1987) diagnosis from the medical record was used to update the computerized drug profile by the facility pharmacist, who also indicated distinctions between drug use for medical and psychiatric purposes after review with physicians or medical records. Diagnoses were classified into one of five groups: 1) schizophrenia (18%), 2) affective disorders (16%), 3) adjustment/personality disorders (24%), 4) conduct disorders (36%), and 5) organic mental disorders (6%).

During the index admission, 11 patients received no psychotropic prescriptions, resulting in a 98% period prevalence of medicated patients ($N = 490$). This population of medicated patients was further refined for purposes of the study to reflect differences by length of stay. The final study group ($N = 330$) had a male-to-female ratio of 3:2 and was divided into short stay (length of stay less than 90 days) ($N = 206$) and long stay (length of stay greater than 90 days) ($N = 124$). Patients receiving prn only orders ($N = 44$) were excluded from the scheduled drug utilization analyses. In addition, 19 patients with diagnoses of organic mental disorders were excluded from further analysis, resulting in a final cohort of 267 patients (60% male).

A prescribing "window" was established consisting of drug records for the first month after admission for short-stay patients or January 1–31, 1990, for long-stay patients, the latter representing prescriptions after a *minimum* length of stay of 90 days. One month of drug data was selected to provide a sufficiently wide interval to capture the variability in drug selection and dosing. Psychotropic drugs were categorized into seven classes according to the American Hospital Formulary Service classification, and the remaining eighth class consisted of miscellaneous agents for psychotropic usage (e.g., carbamazepine, propranolol). Neuroleptic drug dose was expressed as chlorpromazine-equivalent (CPZ-EQ) dose using previously published conversion factors (Baldessarini 1985). The mean total daily dose for patients receiving high-potency agents was compared with that of patients receiving low- to moderate-potency agents. The 11 patients prescribed antipsychotics were classified as either the high-potency group (fluphenazine, haloperidol, thiothixene, trifluoperazine, and pimozide) or the low/moderate-potency group (chlorpromazine, thioridazine, mesoridazine, molindone, perphenazine, and chlorprothixene).

Univariate analyses examined the distribution of males and females according to each of the following variables: age, diagnosis, length of hospitalization, and neuroleptic potency group. Then the frequency of males and females with scheduled psychotropic agents was examined by drug class within the four diagnostic groups. The continuity correction for 2×2 tables was used to adjust for the continuity of the chi-square distribution (Fienberg 1977) and results in a statistic analogous to the Fisher's exact test for small sample sizes. For the neuroleptic-treated patients ($N = 135$), based on the univariate findings, a two-factor analysis of variance (ANOVA) was performed with diagnosis and gender as factors, age as a covariate, and total daily neuroleptic dosage as the dependent variable. The model permits an examination of the neuroleptic daily dose as a function of gender while accounting for the influence of potentially confounding nonpharmacological factors such as diagnosis and age.

Results

Univariate Analyses

Patients' ages were categorized into young (5–12 years), intermediate (13–15 years), and older (16–18 years). The relationship of gender to age indicated significantly more males than females in the 5- to 12-year-old group (71% versus 29%, respectively; $\chi^2 = 9.65$, 2 df, $P < .01$). This difference was also observed in the significantly greater mean age for females (females, 13.7 ± 2.4; males, 13.0 ± 2.9; $t = 2.05$, 254.2 df, $P < .04$). Based on these results, age was included in all subsequent analyses. Diagnostic groups differed according to gender. Whereas patients with conduct disorder were more often male than female (76% versus 24%, respectively; $\chi^2 = 18.41$, 3 df, $P < .0001$), females were nearly twice as frequent in the affective and anxiety/adjustment disorder groups. As with age, diagnosis was shown to be a variable that should be entered into the subsequent ANOVA. However, when gender was related to length of hospitalization, no difference was found ($\chi^2_{\text{cont. corr.}} = 0.6$, 1 df, NS). For this reason, the length of hospital stay was not added to the neuroleptic dosing model.

Psychotropic Drug Utilization

Table 2–1 illustrates the proportions of female and male patients receiving regularly scheduled medications ($N = 267$) according to the eight drug classes. The data indicate that neuroleptics were the most commonly prescribed agents ($N = 135$, 51%). Gender differences for neuroleptic usage were significant: 43% of females compared with 56% of males were medicated with these agents ($\chi^2_{\text{cont. corr.}} = 4.1$, 1 df, $P < .05$). Most striking is the considerable usage across both genders of neuroleptics regardless of the diagnosis. For example, only 33% of the neuroleptic usage is explained by a diagnosis of schizophrenia. The remaining recipients were divided as follows: conduct disorders (36%), affective disorders (21%), and adjustment/personality disorders (10%). Nearly twice as many of the males with conduct disorder received a neuroleptic as their female counterparts (56% versus 30%, respectively; $\chi^2_{\text{cont. corr.}} = 3.7$, 1 df, $P < .06$). Within neuroleptic-treated patients, anticholinergic usage was relatively common, with approximately half of the females and 35% of the males receiving a neuroleptic. Overall, the use of anticholinergic agents along with neuroleptics was not affected by the length of treatment. There was more lithium used as an ancillary agent in males with schizophrenia than in females with this diagnosis (23% versus 4%, respectively), although this was not statistically significant. In the opposite direction, 17% of females with schizophrenia received antidepressants, whereas no males with schizophrenia received this drug class. Finally, stimulant usage in males with conduct disorder was four times greater than in females (18% versus 4%, respectively), whereas the use of miscellaneous agents for psychotropic indications occurred in 8% of females and 9% of males.

Neuroleptic Dosing Patterns

Low-potency neuroleptic agents were prescribed four times more frequently than high-potency agents. However, the selection was

Table 2–1. Frequency of psychotropic drug classes for the cohort of 267 patients with scheduled medications according to gender and diagnostic category

	Females								Males							
	Schizo-phrenia (*N* = 24)		Affective disorders (*N* = 35)		Adjust-ment/personality disorders (*N* = 26)		Conduct dis-orders (*N* = 23)		Schizo-phrenia (*N* = 31)		Affective disorders (*N* = 34)		Adjust-ment/personality disorders (*N* = 21)		Conduct disorders (*N* = 73)	
Drug class	***n***	**%**	***n***	**%**	***n***	**%**	***n***	**%**	***n***	**%**	***n***	**%**	***n***	**%**	***n***	**%**
Neuroleptics[a]	21	88	13	37	5	19	7	30	23	74	16	47	9	43	41	56
Anticholinergics	10	42	8	23	3	12	2	9	15	48	1	3	2	10	13	18
Lithium	1	4	7	20	1	4	5	22	7	23	9	26	—	—	9	12
Antidepressants	4	17	6	17	2	8	4	17	—	—	12	35	1	5	12	16
Anxiolytics/hypnotics	—	—	3	9	2	8	5	22	3	10	4	12	2	10	5	7
Anticonvulsants	2	8	4	11	2	8	2	9	3	10	2	6	1	5	5	7
Stimulants	—	—	—	—	1	4	1	4	1	3	—	—	1	5	13	18
Miscellaneous	1	4	4	11	2	8	1	4	6	19	3	9	1	5	5	7

[a]Neuroleptic usage was significantly greater among males compared with females ($P < .05$).

not affected by gender ($\chi^2_{\text{cont. corr.}}$ = 2.15, 1 df, NS). For this reason, potency group was not entered into the subsequent analyses. Taken as a whole, the cohort received an average dose of 365 ± 515 CPZ-EQ mg/day, with a range of 7–4,567 mg and a median dose of 203 CPZ-EQ mg/day. Overall, females received average total daily doses of neuroleptics that did *not* differ significantly from their male counterparts (339 ± 340 versus 378 ± 586 CPZ-EQ mg/day, respectively, F = 0.61, 1 df, NS) and, by itself, does not support a neuroleptic dosing differential by gender. However, as illustrated in Table 2–2, when the gender groups are split according to diagnostic category, there is a significantly greater daily dosage observed in males with schizophrenia, after accounting for age differences. Based on the two-factor ANOVA results, there is an overall significant effect (F = 3.90, 8 df, P < .001) for differences in neuroleptic dose when diagnosis and gender are factors and age is a covariate. In this model, age explains differences in dosing (F = 5.16, 1 df, P < .02), and, although diagnosis was not significant, there was a diagnosis-by-gender interaction effect (F = 3.00, 1 df, P < .04). The latter effect was observed by post hoc comparison data showing the threefold greater daily dosing of male schizophrenic patients compared with their female counterparts (794 ± 991 mg versus 282 ± 248 CPZ-EQ mg).

Table 2–2. Average total daily dose of neuroleptic expressed in chlorpromazine-equivalents for 46 females and 89 males according to diagnostic group and with age as a covariate in the model

Diagnostic category	Females		Males	
	N	**Mean ± SD**	***N***	**Mean ± SD**
Schizophrenia [a]	21	243 ± 105	23	738 ± 102
Affective disorders	13	395 ± 132	16	354 ± 119
Adjustment/personality disorders	5	292 ± 213	9	278 ± 163
Conduct disorders	7	362 ± 180	41	241 ± 78

[a]Neuroleptic dosage, expressed as average total daily dose in mg chlorpromazine-equivalents, was significantly greater among males with schizophrenia than among females with schizophrenia (P < .001).

Discussion

The influence of gender on neuroleptic usage was considered in this study by utilizing a pharmacoepidemiological data set that focused on the relationship between length of hospitalization and psychotropic usage. The present findings describe gender effects in relation to two outcome measures: neuroleptic selection and neuroleptic dosage. In regard to the first issue, the frequency of neuroleptic selection initially appeared to be influenced by gender, but the observed differences were explained by diagnosis. Thus, although significantly more males received neuroleptics, the result is attributable to the greater proportion of males with conduct disorders, a diagnosis with a male preponderance for neuroleptic treatment in this study. Admittedly, basic questions about the appropriateness and effectiveness of neuroleptics in conduct disorders cannot be addressed by the current data because symptoms and behaviors that might necessitate neuroleptic usage are not available. However, this finding raises several relevant questions for future investigation. For example, did patients with a conduct disorder diagnosis also exhibit attention-deficit/hyperactivity disorder? If so, then a more appropriate pharmacotherapy may involve at least a trial of stimulant medication, given the demonstrated superiority of methylphenidate to the neuroleptic thioridazine for the latter diagnosis (Gittelman-Klein 1992). Such a course of action might be further supported by the relatively high rates of dyskinesias reported among children and adolescents (Campbell et al. 1983) and Gittelman-Klein's assertion that stimulants are the treatment of choice for attention-deficit/hyperactivity disorder.

On the other hand, several textbooks refer to the use of neuroleptics for the diagnosis of conduct disorder (Campbell et al. 1985; Green 1991). This course of action is further supported by findings that schizophrenia was the most common discharge diagnosis among psychiatrically hospitalized adolescents initially diagnosed as conduct disorder (Lewis et al. 1984). In that sample, males with this diagnosis had high rates of paranoid ideation (50%) and psychotic symptoms (55%), both of which might justify neuroleptic intervention. Thus, although the finding of extensive neuroleptic prescription for conduct disorder, especially among male patients, would appear to be questionably justified, further data are needed regarding the symptomatology for which these drugs were used before such a judgment can be made. At a minimum, the trend toward greater neuroleptic use among males in this diagnostic category suggests that gender-specific approaches to such prescription exist although the reasons for this phenomenon are unclear. Nonpharmacological issues that might account for the gender difference include perceived or real propensity for more aggressive behaviors or a greater severity of these behaviors among males than females.

In regard to the second issue of neuroleptic dosing, gender appears to have played a minor role in explaining differences. Our previous findings support length of hospitalization as a factor in explaining neuroleptic dosing (Zito et al. 1988). However, when we examined gender by length of hospitalization, the differences were not significant, whereas age and diagnosis differed. Thus, our ANOVA model entered diagnosis along with gender as factors and included age as a covariate. A significant effect was found for age, but diagnosis played a limited role. Specifically, a diagnosis-by-gender interaction occurred in which males with a diagnosis of schizophrenia were prescribed threefold *greater* daily doses of neuroleptics than females with schizophrenia. Although the present data do not permit us to rule out other nonpharmacological alternative explanations of this observation (e.g., gender-based differences in prescribing physicians' preference and/or symptom pattern or severity), the data suggest the possibility that dosing differences by gender do exist and remain to be explained.

In comparing the findings of this study with those among adult inpatients (Zito et al. 1987), overall average daily doses in this cohort were considerably lower than doses we have measured in adults (mean, 292 ± 337 CPZ-EQ mg/day versus 1,428 ± 1,260 CPZ-EQ mg/day, respectively). Gender was not an issue in regard to the selection of neuroleptic according to its relative potency. Low-potency agents were more frequently used than high-potency agents among both male and female patients, despite recommendations in the pediatric psychopharmacology literature that high-potency agents may be preferable (Campbell and Spencer 1988). The neuroleptic dosing pattern whereby high-potency agents are used at relatively higher doses than low-potency agents, previously described for adult inpatients (Baldessarini et al. 1984; Zito et al. 1987), was found in this study as well, with high-potency agents prescribed at approximately twice the doses of low-potency agents (618 mg versus 294 mg, respectively). Whether this dose differential represents a "ceiling" due to side effects of low-potency agents, a lack of prescribers' knowledge of the relative potency differences, excess dosing of high-potency agents, or a greater relative effectiveness for low-potency agents cannot be ascertained from the current data. Although several of these issues would be costly to resolve, increasing awareness about neuroleptic relative potencies among prescribing physicians is an easy goal to achieve. These findings taken together suggest that child and adolescent psychiatric inpatients are "protected" from exposure to high-dose neuroleptic treatment seen among adult inpatients largely because of the relatively greater predilection for their prescribers to select low-potency neuroleptics. Should current recommendations regarding the preferability of high-potency neuroleptics for this patient population (Campbell and Spencer 1988) be implemented by these prescribers, it remains to be seen whether average daily doses would correspondingly increase as has been the case in adults with, presumably, a concomitant increased risk for long-term adverse effects such as tardive dyskinesia.

Our findings from the previous study of this child/adolescent cohort (Zito et al. 1994) led us to a conceptual model for the selection of neuroleptics that would include, in addition to age and neuroleptic-potency group, diagnosis and length of hospitalization because both factors were significant in explaining differences in the frequency of neuroleptic usage. The implications of increasing dosage and use of neuroleptics over time are far reaching, particularly for the child/adolescent population. Several alternative explanations of the phenomenon need to be explored. First, drug tolerance may occur, although data on this phenomenon in humans are suggestive rather than definitive (Baldessarini 1990). Second, behavioral toxicity (i.e., increased dosage of neuroleptic in response to a worsening of psychotic or behavioral symptoms) may further worsen the behavioral response (Campbell et al. 1985). Third, dosage may be increased when the rate of recovery is slow.

The present study was undertaken to consider whether gender might play a role in this model. When the data were examined by gender, the effect of length of hospitalization did not differ by gender, and thus we constructed an ANOVA model with diagnosis and gender as factors and age as a covariate. Surprisingly, with age in the model, diagnosis assumed a less important role. In fact, diagnosis differed by gender only as an interaction effect: for the male patients with schizophrenia, the average daily dose of neuroleptic was threefold greater than for females with this diagnosis, whereas gender-diagnosis differences did not occur for the other diagnoses. In addition, although when we examine diagnosis alone we find that it explains differences in daily neuroleptic dosing, when age is added to the model, there is little additional dosing difference explained by diagnosis. In summary, the findings of these two studies suggest that a neuroleptic dosing model for children and adolescents should include age, diagnosis, length of hospitalization, and gender. A larger cohort is needed to explore dosing differential for prepubertal versus pubertal females with prospective clinical determination of puberty status if the crucial question of the relationship of estrogens to neuroleptic dosing is to be addressed in child and adolescent psychopharmacology.

The present data suggest directions for future studies of neuroleptic usage in children and adolescents in the usual practice setting. An initial step should be to rule out prescriber differences by developing a protocol for drug selection and dosing changes according to clinical indicators. This would reduce the possibility that drug and dose effects are due to nonspecific factors such as the prescribing physician's preference (Honigfeld 1964; Lehmann 1968; Simeon 1991). Second, the addition of prospectively rated target symptoms and global improvement measures would allow temporal patterns of symptoms and functioning in relation to drug therapy to be more clearly observed and to override expectancy bias in recognizing beneficial effects under conditions in which blinding is not possible. Third, diagnostic criteria should be specified in a more systematic manner than uncontrolled studies permit using structured interviews where possible. Fourth, treatment resistance should be defined so that the impact of medications used for unlabeled indications to augment or replace first-line treatments might be scientifically evaluated. Finally, the relationship between behavioral side effects, drug regimen, and target symptoms should be prospectively and systematically recorded so that behavioral toxicity can be ruled out.

Apart from these research issues, the present findings raise specific questions regarding the risk and effectiveness of current clinical prescribing practices in settings such as those examined in this report. The widespread use of neuroleptics across several diagnostic categories, especially among long-stay patients, raises concern for the development of both short- and long-term movement disorders. The few studies of such disorders among child and adolescent patients have demonstrated a high prevalence of neuroleptic-induced Parkinson-like symptoms that were associated with considerable morbidity (Richardson et al. 1991). The same study indicated a 12% prevalence of treatment-emergent tardive dyskinesia among patients receiving neuroleptics for more than 3 months, with more females than males exhibiting this side effect despite a marked predominance of male patients in the total study sample. If it can be assumed that many of these children and adolescent patients are at high risk for continued or intermittent exposure to neuroleptics over a lifetime, then concern is raised by the current data indicating the use of these agents across a broad diagnostic spectrum, including diagnoses not usually considered to be indications for their use among adult patients.

The focus of the present report is on gender-specific prescribing practices and their clinical implications. In this regard, female patients appeared to be at somewhat less risk of receiving neuroleptics for unlabeled indications than male patients. In addition, among patients with schizophrenia, the average daily neuroleptic dose was significantly lower among female patients. Both findings suggest a somewhat more clinically restrained approach to the prescription of these drugs among young women inpatients. This finding is encouraging given recent evidence of increased vulnerability of women to both endocrine (Zito et al. 1990) and extrapyramidal side effects of neuroleptic medication (Yassa and Jeste 1992). The latter report was a literature review that found women to show a higher prevalence of tardive dyskinesia and more severe tardive dyskinesia than men, particularly in the postmenopausal age range. Further, it has been suggested (Seeman 1983) that a gender-by-age-by-neuroleptic interaction effect occurs in which endogenous estrogens may protect premenopausal women from developing tardive dyskinesia via their antidopaminergic activity (Raymond et al. 1978), either directly (Villeneuve et al. 1980) or by enabling the use of lower neuroleptic doses. The present findings are relevant to these observations in several ways. First, the current sample size and the absence of clinical data regarding pubertal status of the study subjects prevent our examination of the findings in relation to estrogen effect. However, if the above suggestions regarding a "protective" estrogen effect are valid, then prepubertal female patients might be at equally increased risk of neuroleptic-induced side effects such as tardive dyskinesia as their postmenopausal sisters. Clearly, clinical studies are needed to explore the implications of such a possibility.

Conversely, our observation that female patients with diagnoses of schizophrenia received significantly lower average daily doses of neuroleptic than their male counterparts is consistent with the antidopaminergic effect of estrogens in reducing the need for neuroleptics among postpubertal females (Seeman 1986). From this finding, we might predict that the majority of females with a diagnosis of schizophrenia in this study had passed into puberty. On the other hand, the fact that there was no essential gender difference in average daily dose of neuroleptic among patients with nonschizophrenic diagnoses and the fact that females received nonsignificantly higher doses than males in these cases raise questions about either the hormonal status or effectiveness of drugs in these patient populations. Two main possibilities emerge from this discussion: either most females in the nonschizophrenic diagnostic categories did not experience the estrogenic antidopaminergic effect (i.e., were prepubertal), or the drugs were equally effective or ineffective for both gender groups. If the former were true, then there would be a concern for these patients being at increased risk for developing tardive dyskinesia; if the latter were true, then either all patients would be seen as inappropriately at risk for neuroleptic side effects or the postulated estrogen effect is specific for schizophrenia. Clearly, further studies, either clinically controlled or naturalistic studies such as those described above, are needed to address these issues.

Finally, if the assumption can be made that the use of neuroleptics in this patient population is effective across diagnostic categories, the present findings raise concerns about compliance with continued treatment, which may also be gender specific. Prior studies (Richardson et al. 1991) have shown that the presence of Parkinson-like side effects is associated with self-reports of noncompliance with drug therapy among child and adolescent patients. Because such side effects tend to be dose related and often are ameliorated by anticholinergic agents, the male patients with schizophrenia in the present study would appear to be at greater risk given their significantly higher average daily dose of neuroleptics; likewise, male patients in other diagnostic categories would seem to be at high risk for such symptoms given their low exposure to anticholinergic drugs relative to their exposure to neuroleptics.

Because high-potency neuroleptic agents appear to have a higher propensity for the induction of prolactin response than low-potency agents (Langer et al. 1977; Zito et al. 1990), postpubertal female patients in this study were less likely to be vulnerable to noncompliance secondary to the emergence of these effects given the fourfold difference in the use of low- versus high-potency agents. In all these cases, a clinical prospective study would be needed to determine which doses and potency agents are most effective in minimizing side effects likely to interfere with compliance with outpatient treatment.

References

Adams S: Prescribing of psychotropic drugs to children and adolescents [see comments]. BMJ 302:217, 1991

American Psychiatric Association: Diagnostic and Statistical Manual of Mental Disorders, 3rd Edition, Revised. Washington, DC, American Psychiatric Association, 1987

American Psychiatric Association: Tardive Dyskinesia: A Task Force Report of the American Psychiatric Association. Washington, DC, American Psychiatric Association, 1992

Baldessarini RJ: Chemotherapy in Psychiatry: Principles and Practice, 2nd Edition. Cambridge, MA, Harvard University Press, 1985

Baldessarini RJ: Drugs and the treatment of psychiatric disorders, in Goodman and Gilman's Pharmacological Basis of Therapeutics, 8th Edition. Edited by Gilman AG, Rall TW, Nies AS, et al. New York, Macmillan, 1990, pp 383–435

Baldessarini RJ, Katz B, Cotton P: Dissimilar dosing with high-potency and low-potency neuroleptics. Am J Psychiatry 141:748–752, 1984

Biederman J: New developments in pediatric psychopharmacology. J Am Acad Child Adolesc Psychiatry 31:14–15, 1992

Campbell M, Spencer EK: Psychopharmacology in child and adolescent psychiatry: a review of the past five years. J Am Acad Child Adolesc Psychiatry 27:269–279, 1988

Campbell M, Grega DM, Green WH, et al: Neuroleptic-induced dyskinesias in children. Clin Neuropharmacol 6:207–222, 1983

Campbell M, Green WH, Deutsch SI: Child and Adolescent Psychopharmacology. Beverly Hills, CA, Sage, 1985

Chouinard G, Annable L, Steinberg S: A controlled clinical trial of fluspirilene, a long-acting injectable neuroleptic, in schizophrenic patients with acute exacerbation. J Clin Psychopharmacol 6:21–26, 1986

Collins PJ, Larkin EP, Shubsachs AP: Lithium carbonate in chronic schizophrenia: a brief trial of lithium carbonate added to neuroleptics for treatment of resistant schizophrenic patients. Acta Psychiatr Scand 84:150–154, 1991

Cooperstock R: Sex differences in the use of mood-modifying drugs: an explanatory model. J Health Soc Behav 12:238–244, 1971

Craig TJ, Van Natta PA: Current medication use and symptoms of depression in a general population. Am J Psychiatry 135:1036–1039, 1978

Elliger TJ, Trott GE, Nissen G: Prevalence of psychotropic medication in childhood and adolescence in the Federal Republic of Germany. Pharmacopsychiatry 23:38–44, 1990

Ereshefsky L, Saklad SR, Watanabe MD, et al: Thiothixene pharmacokinetic interactions: a study of hepatic enzyme inducers, clearance inhibitors, and demographic variables [published erratum appears in J Clin Psychopharmacol 12:78, 1992]. J Clin Psychopharmacol 11:296–301, 1991

Fienberg SE: The Analysis of Cross-Classified Data. Cambridge, MA, MIT Press, 1977

Gittelman-Klein R: Pharmacotherapy of childhood hyperactivity: an update, in Psychopharmacology: The Third Generation of Progress. Edited by Meltzer HY. New York, Raven, 1992, pp 1215–1224

Green WH: Child and Adolescent Clinical Psychopharmacology. Baltimore, MD, Williams & Wilkins, 1991

Hohmann AA: Gender bias in psychotropic drug prescribing in primary care. Med Care 27:478–490, 1989

Honigfeld G: Non-specific factors in treatment. Diseases of the Nervous System 25:225–239, 1964

Jatlow PI: Psychotropic drug disposition during development, in Psychiatric Pharmacosciences of Children and Adolescents. Edited by Popper C. Washington, DC, American Psychiatric Press, 1987, pp 29–44

Langer G, Sachar EJ, Gruen PH, et al: Human prolactin responses to neuroleptic drugs correlate with antischizophrenic potency. Nature 266:639–640, 1977

Lehmann HE: Problems in controlled clinical evaluations, in Psychopharmacology: A Review of Progress 1957–1967. Edited by Efron DH. Washington, DC, U.S. Government Printing Office, 1968, pp 949–971

Lewis DO, Lewis M, Unger L, et al: Conduct disorder and its synonyms: diagnoses of dubious validity and usefulness. Am J Psychiatry 141:514–519, 1984

Parry HJ, Balter MB, Mellinger GD, et al: National patterns of psychotherapeutic drug use. Arch Gen Psychiatry 28:18–74, 1973

Quinn DMP: Prevalence of psychoactive medication in children and adolescents. Can J Psychiatry 31:575–580, 1986

Raymond V, Beaulieu M, Labrie F, et al: Potent antidopaminergic activity of estradiol at the pituitary level on prolactin release. Science 200:1173–1175, 1978

Richardson MA, Haugland G, Craig TJ: Neuroleptic use, parkinsonian symptoms, tardive dyskinesia, and associated factors in child and adolescent psychiatric patients. Am J Psychiatry 148:1322–1328, 1991

Seeman MV: Interaction of sex, age, and neuroleptic dose. Compr Psychiatry 24:125–128, 1983

Seeman MV: Current outcome in schizophrenia: women vs men. Acta Psychiatr Scand 73:609–617, 1986

Simeon JG: Pediatric psychopharmacology. Can J Psychiatry 34:115–122, 1989

Simeon JG: Child psychopharmacology. J Am Acad Child Adolesc Psychiatry 30:695–696, 1991

Simpson GM, Yadalam KG, Levinson DF, et al: Single-dose pharmacokinetics of fluphenazine after fluphenazine decanoate administration. J Clin Psychopharmacol 10:417–421, 1990

Teicher MH, Baldessarini RJ: Developmental pharmacodynamics, in Psychiatric Pharmacosciences of Children and Adolescents. Edited by Popper C. Washington, DC, American Psychiatric Press, 1987, pp 45–80

Villeneuve A, Cazejust T, Cote M: Estrogens in tardive dyskinesia in male psychiatric patients. Neuropsychobiology 6:145–151, 1980

Waters BGH: Psychopharmacology of the psychiatric disorders of childhood and adolescence. Therapeutics 152:32–39, 1990

Yassa R, Jeste DV: Gender differences in tardive dyskinesia: a critical review of the literature. Schizophr Bull 18:701–715, 1992

Yonkers KA, Kando JC, Cole JO, et al: Gender differences in pharmacokinetics and pharmacodynamics of psychotropic medication. Am J Psychiatry 149:587–595, 1992

Young MA, Meltzer HY: The relationship of demographic, clinical, and outcome variables to neuroleptic treatment requirements. Schizophr Bull 6:88–101, 1980

Zito JM, Craig TJ, Wanderling J, et al: Pharmaco-epidemiology in 136 hospitalized schizophrenic patients. Am J Psychiatry 144:778–782, 1987

Zito JM, Craig TJ, Wanderling J, et al: Pharmacotherapy of the hospitalized young adult schizophrenic patient. Compr Psychiatry 29:379–386, 1988

Zito JM, Sofair JB, Jaeger J: Self-reported neuroendocrine effects of antipsychotics in women: a pilot study. DICP 24:176–180, 1990

Zito JM, Craig TJ, Wanderling J: Pharmacoepidemiology of 330 child/adolescent psychiatric patients. Journal of Pharmacoepidemiology 3:47–62, 1994

CHAPTER 3

Typicality and Atypicality in the Development of Neuroleptic Side Effects in Child and Adolescent Psychiatric Patients

Mary Ann Richardson, Ph.D.
Gary Haugland, M.A.

Since the first reports of the neurological side effects of neuroleptics began to appear in the early 1950s, clinicians have sought to minimize these side effects without sacrificing therapeutic efficacy. The emergence of side effects in patients compromises their well-being not only by threatening treatment compliance but by introducing a somatic stressor that carries with it the potential for worsening psychiatric status. On the part of clinicians, the fear of inducing side effects in their patients creates a psychological cap on the neuroleptic dose range they administer. This cap often keeps the dose below the level of achievable treatment efficacy, thus cheating patients and their families of the full benefit of available psychiatric treatment. In no field has this psychological cap been more palpable as in the field of child and adolescent psychopharmacology.

In our work we have sought to define in the major neuroleptic-treated populations both the extent and seriousness of certain neurological side effects—parkinsonism (PK) and tardive dyskinesia (TD)—and, with an eye to prevention, to establish clinically recognizable risk factors for the disorders. In one such investigation in children and adolescents who were psychiatric inpatients (Richardson et al. 1991), we reported on four patients that we followed over a period of time. This longitudinal look allowed us to see an atypicality in the relationship between changes in medication status and PK and/or TD status. The atypicality issue had been unexpected and emerged from the study data in the course of the analyses.

Individual case atypicality refers to the deviation in observed movement disorder status from the expected movement disorder response to changes in the patient's medication status. The primary expected movement disorder responses are outlined in Table 3–1. For instance, it is expected that for most patients, an increase in neuroleptic dose will result in a decrease in TD symp-

Table 3–1. Criterion symptoms for parkinsonism designation and tardive dyskinesia designation

Parkinsonism scale items[a]
Gait—stiff, shuffling, stooped
Arms—diminished swing and resistance to free fall
Shoulders, elbows, wrists—stiffness, rigidity, resistance to movement
Legs—resistance to swing
Neck—rigidity, resistance to free fall
Tremor—primarily resting
Salivation—excess, pooling
Glabellar tap response—abnormal
Tardive dyskinesia items included in global score[b]
Puckering, smacking lip movements
Chewing and lateral jaw movements
Bonbon sign—tongue pushing against cheeks or upper or lower lip
Tongue protrusion
Choreoathetoid movements of the tongue
Cheek puffing
Axial hyperkinesia—pelvic thrusting
Choreoathetoid movements of fingers, wrists, ankles, and toes

[a]Total score of 4 or more.
[b]Global score of mild to severe.

tom levels and an increase in PK symptom levels. These norms have been formulated almost exclusively from clinical and research experience in adult populations.

Beyond the individual case atypicality of these four case studies, we also saw a deviation from the adult literature in the primary study findings of a 34% prevalence of PK and a 12% prevalence of TD (treatment emergent). These prevalence data contrasted with our findings in adult populations in which the same instruments and case criteria were used as in the child/adolescent investigation. For instance, a lower prevalence of PK (24%) was seen in a sample of psychiatric inpatients, ages 25–34 (Richardson 1989; Richardson et al. 1989a), and a higher prevalence of TD (58%) was seen in a large adult inpatient population (Richardson et al. 1989c).

In the interests of providing the treating clinician with information that has not heretofore been available, for the present chapter we have focused on this issue of individual case atypicality and have expanded the number of cases studied over time from 4 to 10. This has allowed us a more intense look at the issue of how children and adolescents deviate from the expected norms of the response of PK and TD symptoms to changes in medication. Our methods, which are defined below, were to study individual child and adolescent patients with these side effects over multiple evaluations.

Methods

The study pool for the initial study had consisted of all children and adolescents who were residents at a New York State Office of Mental Health Children's Psychiatric Center at the onset of the study or admitted during the following 6 months. All residents were evaluated as a clinical procedure, and consent was obtained from parents or guardians for the research use of the data. Verbal assent was obtained from all patients as well, prior to their participation in the neurological evaluation.

Most recent diagnoses were collected from the patients' facility charts. Behavioral characteristics (history of alcohol abuse, drug abuse, stealing, arson, assaultiveness, suicide attempts, hyperactivity, running away) and factors of family history (physical or sexual abuse, history of psychiatric hospitalization among first-degree relatives) were extracted from the patients' charts both at the study facility and from records collected during prior admissions at other facilities.

The patients were rated for TD by means of the Simpson Abbreviated Dyskinesia Scale (Simpson et al. 1979) and for PK using the Simpson-Angus Neurological Rating Scale (Simpson and Angus 1970). Subjects were evaluated using a 23-step movement disorder rating procedure lasting approximately 45 minutes per patient that was designed to maximize the validity of the differential diagnosis by including activities that had been tested to increase and diminish movement counts. The reliability of the rating procedures has been previously reported (Richardson et al. 1986b). Patients were also interviewed as to their assessment of the efficacy of their treatment and their view of their side effect experience.

The presence of PK was defined by a minimum total score of 4 from items 1–10 of the Neurological Rating Scale. The symptoms that are included in that designation are defined in Table 3–1. TD criterion measures were based on a consensual clinical diagnosis from simultaneous evaluations by the two raters derived from the Abbreviated Dyskinesia Scale global score rating of mild to severe, a method that has been reported previously (Richardson and Casey 1988; Richardson and Craig 1982; Richardson et al. 1984, 1985, 1986a, 1986b, 1989b). The abnormal movements that were the criterion for the TD-yes designation are listed in Table 3–1. Raters were kept blind to medication status, diagnosis, and psychiatric treatment history.

Subsequent to the rating, neuroleptic treatment histories were collected from a computerized information system at the inpatient facility and records obtained from the patients' first treating facility and facilities the patient had been in immediately preceding the current admission. Only medication received while the patients were in residence in a facility were included for analysis because the interviews we held with the patients revealed a high rate of out-of-hospital noncompliance.

TD and PK were assessed at each of the rating sessions, and the changes in scores became the basis of the following case reports and thus the core data of this chapter. Medication use data were studied for the period from 30 days prior to rating 1 and for every day in between up to the day of the last rating (either rating 2 or 3). The neuroleptic and antiparkinson use variables that were reviewed as being associated with changes in PK and TD status were: 1) chlorpromazine-equivalent (CPZ-EQ) dose at time of evaluation (a listing of these equivalences for common neuroleptics is found in Table 3–2), 2) anticholinergic equivalent activity at

Table 3–2. Chlorpromazine equivalency

Generic name	Brand name	Equivalence[a]
Chlorpromazine	Thorazine	100[b]
Prochlorperazine	Compazine	15[b]
Perphenazine	Trilafon	10[b]
Trifluoperazine	Stelazine	5[b]
Thioridazine	Mellaril	100[b]
Acetophenazine	Tindal	25[b]
Butaperazine	Repoise	10[b]
Mesoridazine	Serentil	50[b]
Piperacetazine	Quide	10[b]
Haloperidol	Haldol	2[c]
Chlorprothixene	Taractan	75[c]
Thiothixene	Navane	5[b]
Loxapine	Loxitane	15[c]
Molindone	Moban	10[c]
Amoxapine	Asendin	200[d]
Fluphenazine	Prolixin	2[b]
Fluphenazine decanoate	Prolixin	[e]
	25 mg Q1W	1,000 CPZ-EQ/day
	25 mg Q2W	500 CPZ-EQ/day
	25 mg Q3W	332 CPZ-EQ/day

[a]Dose required to achieve therapeutic efficacy of 100 mg of chlorpromazine.
[b]Davis 1985.
[c]Baldessarini 1985.
[d]J. O. Cole, personal communication, November 1985.
[e]T. Cooper, personal communication, November 1985.

time of evaluation (a listing of these equivalences for several classes of drugs is found in Table 3–3), 3) average CPZ-EQ dose in the period immediately prior to the first rating and the time between subsequent ratings, and 4) average anticholinergic activity in these same time frames. The anticholinergic activity factor

Table 3–3. Anticholinergic activity factors (human caudate nucleus)

Generic name	Brand name	Factor value
Chlorpromazine	Thorazine	1.4[a]
Prochlorperazine	Compazine	0.18[a]
Perphenazine	Trilafon	0.067[a]
Trifluoperazine	Stelazine	0.15[a]
Thioridazine	Mellaril	5.6[a]
Mesoridazine	Serentil	1.4[a]
Haloperidol	Haldol	0.0042[a]
Thiothixene	Navane	0.034[a]
Loxapine	Loxitane	0.22[a]
Molindone	Moban	0.00026[a]
Amoxapine	Asendin	0.1[b]
Fluphenazine	Prolixin	0.053[a]
Amitriptyline	Elavil	5.5[b]
Trihexyphenidyl	Artane	30.0[c]
Diphenhydramine	Benadryl	0.91[c]
Clozapine	Clozaril	8.3[a]
Benztropine	Cogentin	80.0[c]
Desipramine	Norpramin	0.5[b]
Doxepin	Sinequan	1.3[b]
Imipramine	Tofranil	1.1[b]
Maprotiline	Ludiomil	0.2[b]
Nortriptyline	Pamelor	0.7[b]

[a]Richelson 1984.
[b]Richelson 1983.
[c]E. Richelson, personal communication, March 1988.

was a sum of the total anticholinergic exposure of the patient, including that exposure that was derived from neuroleptics, antiparkinson agents, and diphenhydramine. Changes occurring across the multiple evaluations were used to determine the typicality and atypicality assessments. Table 3–4 lists the patterns of the response of PK and TD symptoms to medication changes that were considered typical.

The subjects described in this chapter were selected from 22 patients for whom multiple ratings were performed. In the original investigation, multiple ratings were performed on three groups of patients: those who were designated as a positive TD case at their first rating, those who were given a questionable TD rating at their first evaluation, and a random selection of other patients until 20% of the entire sample was reached. The 10 patients discussed in this chapter were those who had received a positive TD and/or PK designation at any rating. The other 12 patients were not included because in 4 cases they had not received neuroleptic medication nor had they developed any side effects, and the remaining 8, although they did receive medication while hospitalized, did not meet the criterion measures for the development of TD or PK side effects at any of their evaluations.

Results

Table 3–5 provides the demographic and behavioral characteristics of the study subjects. As can be seen from a review of the table, the subjects break out evenly by sex; however, the mean age of

Table 3–4. Expected responses to changes in medication status in terms of tardive dyskinesia and parkinsonism symptoms

Change in medication	Tardive dyskinesia	Parkinsonism
Increase in neuroleptic dose	↓	↑
Increase in anticholinergic activity	↑	↓
Decrease in dose or discontinuation of neuroleptic	↑	↓
Decrease in anticholinergic activity	↓	↑

Table 3–5. Demographic and behavioral characteristics of children with multiple ratings

Patient	Gender	Age	Diagnosis	Alcohol abuse	Drug abuse	Stealing
A	Male	15.4	Conduct disorder			
B	Female	14.4	Major depression			
C	Female	17.6	Schizoaffective			
D	Male	17.1	Atypical depression	Y	Y	
E	Female	15.5	Schizophreniform			Y
F	Female	16.0	Conduct disorder		Y	
G	Male	13.6	Adjustment disorder			
H	Female	13.8	Schizophrenia			
I	Male	10.3	Attention-deficit/ hyperactivity disorder			
J	Male	13.3	Conduct disorder			
Total	Females	15.5		0	1	1
	Males	13.9		1	1	0
	All	14.7		10%	20%	10%

Note. Y indicates presence of the characteristic.

the study females is somewhat higher than that for the males. There is a broad range of diagnoses represented; the predominant behavioral characteristic was a history of assaultive behavior (60%), and half of the subjects revealed a history of psychiatric hospitalization among their first-degree relatives.

The data in Table 3–6 provide the basis for the TD and PK typicality and atypicality designations in terms of the relationship between symptom changes and changes in the treatment regimen. The derivation of these designations was more specifically derived from the interaction of the CPZ-EQ data, the anticholin-

Arson	Assaul-tiveness	Suicide attempts	Hyper-activity	Running away	Physical or sexual abuse	Family history
			Y		Y	Y
		Y				Y
	Y			Y		
						Y
Y		Y			Y	Y
	Y			Y		
	Y	Y	Y		Y	
	Y					
	Y		Y		Y	Y
	Y			Y		
1	3	2	0	2	1	2
0	3	1	3	1	3	3
10%	60%	30%	30%	30%	40%	50%

ergic activity profiles, and the pattern of medication use with changes in PK and TD status and severity. As noted earlier, Table 3–2 provides a listing of the equivalences, and Table 3–3 provides the anticholinergic activity profiles that were used; Table 3–1 defines the side effect symptoms that were the criterion for TD and PK designations and severity levels.

What can be seen from a study of Table 3–6 is a wide range of neuroleptic doses and anticholinergic activity exposure. We see no treatment regimens that are particularly associated with the side effects of PK and TD or to alterations in the symptom levels of those disorders. What is seen rather is a heterogeneity in these matters.

Table 3–6. Summary of multiple ratings of child psychiatric patients' chlorpromazine equivalents (CPZ-EQ), anticholinergic activity, tardive dyskinesia (TD), and parkinsonism (PK)

	Patient									
	A	**B**	**C**	**D**	**E**	**F**	**G**	**H**	**I**	**J**
Prior to first rating										
Days (N)	30	9	3	30	30	15	30	30	30	17
CPZ-EQ (mean)	50	100	100	775	233	1,267	49	405	260	400
Anticholinergic (mean)	90	564	80.8	160.5	1.8	160	275.3	1,783	36.6	672.9
First rating										
CPZ -EQ	50	100	100	750	300	1,500	25	300	400	400
Anticholinergic	90	560	80.8	160.8	2.3	160	140	82.3	36.8	640
TD score	8	no	no	no	no	no	no	no	no	no
PK score	no	15	6	7	14	no	17	no	no	no

Between ratings 1 & 2										
Days (*N*)	56	19	45	29	91	128	27	64	90	57[a]
CPZ-EQ (mean)	50	100	417	871	1,102	1,797	50	300	700	296
Anticholinergic (mean)	24.3	720	20.1	136.1	152.2	160	360	25	10.9	447.4
Second rating										
CPZ-EQ	50	100	500	750	1,000	2,000	50	300	800	0
Anticholinergic	10	720	18.2	80.8	160	160	360	2.3	0.9	0
TD score	no	no	no	5	6	6	no	no	no	no
PK score	no	8	no	6	7	4	14	4	8	8
Between ratings 2 & 3										
Days (*N*)	41	16			15[b]		72			
CPZ-EQ (mean)	40	100			433		50			
Anticholinergic (mean)	7.5	720			100		282.2			

(continued)

Table 3–6. Summary of multiple ratings of child psychiatric patients' chlorpromazine equivalents (CPZ-EQ), anticholinergic activity, tardive dyskinesia (TD), and parkinsonism (PK) *(continued)*

	Patient									
	A	B	C	D	E	F	G	H	I	J
Third rating										
CPZ-EQ	38	100			0		50			
Anticholinergic	7.5	720			0		280			
TD score	3	no			11		no			
PK score	no	15			9		11			

[a]Off neuroleptic 8 days before rating.
[b]Off neuroleptic 5 days before rating.

Aside from our focused issue of atypicality, attention should be drawn to the severity of PK symptoms seen in 3 of our 10 patients (B, E, G). The symptom level of patient G is of particular concern because it suggests an acute vulnerability to the manifestation of this side effect in this patient, particularly in light of both the low level of neuroleptic exposure he was experiencing in the evaluation period and the high anticholinergic potency of the neuroleptic (thioridazine) he was receiving. Patient B was also receiving thioridazine throughout the study period. Patient E, although not receiving thioridazine, showed a severe level of TD symptoms at her third rating in addition to the severe PK. This should not be unexpected, however, because she may have been experiencing a withdrawal dyskinesia at that evaluation, her neuroleptic treatment having been discontinued 5 days prior.

The following is a patient-by-patient assessment of the issue of typicality of the pharmacology of PK and TD in our study subjects. As noted, these assessments are derived primarily from the data presented in Table 3–6.

Patient A has been assigned the designation of a typical TD pattern. This adolescent male with a diagnosis of conduct disorder was being treated with amoxapine throughout the evaluation period. He reached a TD-yes criterion level on both his first and his third rating sessions. His TD pattern was typical in that he had his highest TD score at the first rating when he was receiving benztropine and thus experiencing his highest level of anticholinergic exposure.

Patient B demonstrates both a typical and an atypical pattern of PK severity to medication changes. It should be noted that this female adolescent carried a diagnosis of major depression and was one of three patients experiencing a very substantial level of PK symptoms throughout the three evaluations. This severity of symptoms is all the more surprising given the relatively high level of anticholinergic potency in the neuroleptic (thioridazine) that she was being treated with throughout the evaluation period. A typical PK picture was seen in the changes between ratings 1 and 2; an increase in anticholinergic exposure (brought on by a switch from diphenhydramine to benztropine) saw a concomitant decrease of 53% in her total PK score. An atypical PK-medication interaction was seen, however, between ratings 2 and 3 in that her total PK score increased by 88% while she was receiving the same neuroleptic dose and the same dose of benztropine as she was at rating 1.

Patient C, who showed a markedly atypical pattern for her PK symptoms, carried a diagnosis of schizoaffective disorder and received treatment with both trifluoperazine and molindone during the evaluation period. She showed PK only at rating 1 while she was being treated with trifluoperazine and benztropine. At rating 2, she was being treated with a substantially higher CPZ-EQ neuroleptic dose and had been switched from benztropine to diphenhydramine. Her overall PK manifestation was atypical on two counts in that she showed symptoms only at rating 1 when she was both on the lower neuroleptic dose and the higher level of anticholinergic activity.

Patient D showed atypical patterns for both PK and TD. He was treated with both fluphenazine and haloperidol during the evaluation period. Prior to the first rating, he started out on fluphenazine, was switched to haloperidol, then back to fluphenazine, and he continued on fluphenazine through to the second evaluation. He also experienced a decrease in the dose of benztropine between ratings 1 and 2 so that by rating 2 the dose of that drug had been cut in half. At rating 1, this adolescent male, with a diagnosis of atypical depression, showed only symptoms of PK; at rating 2, he showed coexisting TD and PK. The PK was atypical in that, despite an increase in neuroleptic exposure in the month between ratings 1 and 2 and a decrease in anticholinergic exposure, the score severity remained at almost the same level (a total score of 7 versus a total score of 6). The TD emergent pattern was also atypical in that symptoms were seen only at the second rating after the decrease in anticholinergic exposure.

Patient E, an adolescent female with a diagnosis of schizophreniform disorder, showed both substantial symptomatology and typical pharmacology in both disorders. She was treated with both trifluoperazine and molindone during the evaluation period and then had a neuroleptic discontinuation period of 5 days prior to the third rating. In addition to her neuroleptic treatment, she received benztropine both between ratings 1 and 2 and between ratings 2 and 3. She showed coexisting TD and PK at ratings 2 and 3, and PK at all three evaluations. The typicality of her symptom patterns for PK is evidenced by a cutting in half in symptom level with a substantial increase in anticholinergic exposure between ratings 1 and 2. Her TD emerged at the second rating after she had experienced a change in neuroleptic (trifluoperazine to molindone) and a marked increase in dose. The increased dose brought with it a substantial increase in the level of anticholinergic exposure. The assigning of a typical or an atypical classification is quite complex as the increased CPZ-EQ dose would be expected to mask any TD symptoms, whereas the increased anticholinergic exposure from the increased dose in neuroleptic would be expected to aggravate or unmask the TD. The TD symptom picture does show typicality, however, when the symptom severity doubles with a discontinuation of the neuroleptic treatment.

Patient F is an adolescent female who shows typicality for PK but atypicality for TD. She was treated with molindone and a stable dose of benztropine throughout the evaluation period. At the first evaluation, she showed no symptoms of either movement disorder; at the second evaluation, however, both disorders emerged when she experienced an increase in neuroleptic dose. It can be expected that the PK would emerge with the substantial increase in neuroleptic dose; it is not expected, however, that the TD would do so as the higher neuroleptic dose would be expected to mask rather than uncover the TD symptoms.

Patient G is a 13.6-year-old male with a diagnosis of adjustment disorder who shows an atypical PK symptoms to treatment relationship. He was treated with low doses of thioridazine throughout the entire evaluation period and also received benztropine (1 mg) in the period between ratings 1 and 2 and at rating 2. Aside from the issue of typicality, the most predominant feature of the side-effect experience of this patient is the very substantial PK symptoms he experienced throughout the period, all while receiving low doses of neuroleptics. He showed his most severe PK symptomatology after a 30-day period of downward dose titration of his thioridazine (at rating 1) to its lowest level throughout the period; for that reason, we give him a designation of atypicality.

Patient H is an adolescent female with a diagnosis of schizophrenia who shows a typical PK to treatment response. She was treated with thioridazine prior to the first rating and was on trifluoperazine at the first rating. She showed only mild PK and only at rating 2 after more than 2 months on the trifluoperazine (lower anticholinergic activity than thioridazine) and further when she was on amantadine rather than the benztropine she had been treated with at the first rating.

Patient I is a 10-year-old male with a clinical diagnosis of attention-deficit/hyperactivity disorder who shows an atypical PK to treatment pattern. He was treated with haloperidol and diphenhydramine prior to the first rating, with the diphenhydramine continuing to the first rating day; he was on fluphenazine at rating 1 and throughout the period between ratings 1 and 2. The diphenhydramine was discontinued 65 days before rating 2. This patient showed very substantial PK side effects at rating 1, which decreased at rating 2. His pattern of PK symptoms is thus atypical in that he shows a 43% decline in symptoms with a doubling of neuroleptic dose and the discontinuation of diphenhydramine.

Patient J is a 13-year-old male with a clinical diagnosis of conduct disorder who has an atypical PK response. He was treated with a chlorpromazine-benztropine combination prior to the first rating, with the benztropine continuing only up to 34 days before rating 2 and chlorpromazine up to 8 days before rating 2, at which time it too was discontinued. We are defining the PK symptom profile for this patient as atypical because it first manifested itself at rating 2 after a period of lower neuroleptic exposure due to the medication discontinuation.

Table 3–7 presents the summary for the 10 patients of the atypical and typical relationships seen between neurological side effects and pharmacological interventions as we have defined them. We can see thus that atypicality appears to be the norm in that 7 of 10 patients (70%) showed a neuroleptic-induced neurological symptom expression that represents an atypical association with their medication regimen. Further, we can see that this atypicality is more prominent with PK (67%) than TD (50%). To add to the complexity, patient B manifests both typical and atypical PK pharmacology. Most striking, however, is the gender difference seen, with males having nearly twice as many atypical symptom expressions as females (83% versus 43%). The gender difference becomes even more striking when looking at PK alone, with all of the males with PK having an atypical expression versus only 40% of the females.

Table 3–7. Typicality of side effects among children with multiple ratings

	Parkinsonism		Tardive dyskinesia	
Patient	**Typical**	**Atypical**	**Typical**	**Atypical**
A			Y	
B[a]	Y	Y		
C		Y		
D		Y		Y
E	Y		Y	
F	Y			Y
G		Y		
H	Y			
I		Y		
J		Y		

Note. Y indicates whether response was typical or atypical.
[a]Patient B exhibited both typical and atypical responses at different rating sessions.

Discussion

Over the course of these multiple evaluations, we have uncovered an atypicality in the pharmacology of neuroleptic-induced disorders of PK and TD in children and adolescents. This atypicality, one could assume, either arises from a particular vulnerability to develop the disorder so that it emerges or worsens even in atypical situations or there is an inherently different neurochemical substrate for the atypical responses. Although we have seen that the majority of responses in the symptoms of the disorders of PK and TD to changes in the medication mix are atypical, we have also seen that this atypicality is more predominant for neuroleptic-induced PK, a disorder that has been given scant attention in the fields of both adult and child psychopharmacology (Richardson et al. 1991).

Furthermore, we see gender differences in side-effect typicality for PK, an area in which, as far as we know, no work has been done in children and very little in adults. These gender findings were most striking in that all of the males with PK showed atypical patterns of symptom response to changes in the treatment regimen, whereas for the females it was only those with affective components to their illnesses who showed atypical PK pharmacology (patient B with a diagnosis of major depression and patient C with a diagnosis of schizoaffective disorder). What also emerges in the data is an interaction between diagnosis and age; among our male patients, the only one older than 13.6 years who showed an atypical PK pharmacology is also carrying an affective disorder diagnosis (atypical depression).

Explanation of these findings leads us to several other areas of work. In terms of a particular vulnerability for PK in patients with affective symptomatology, as seen in our cases, there have been a number of reports in the adult psychopharmacology literature showing significant statistical associations between affective symptomatology and neuroleptic-induced PK status and severity in psychiatric patients (Craig et al. 1985; Galdi 1983; Johnson 1981; Richardson et al. 1988). We can thus suggest that our adolescent females were vulnerable to PK atypicality only when they carried the extra vulnerability of a neurochemical substrate that leads to affective illness.

In terms of the male vulnerability to atypical PK being seen primarily in the boys under age 14, some other large-scale epidemiological work we have done (Richardson 1989; Richardson et al. 1989a) across ages 8–85 has demonstrated that the vulnerability to the development of PK is most acute in the age ranges of prepubertal adolescents and patients over 65. These findings for the PK life cycle may be related to interactions between sex hormones and the enzyme monoamine oxidase. Monoamine oxidase is relevant to our concerns about neuroleptic-induced PK as its function is the oxidative deamination of the monoaminergic neurotransmitter, dopamine, and hypodopaminergia is a necessary neurochemical substrate for neuroleptic-induced PK. It is known that the activity of monoamine oxidase is affected by the activity of the sex hormones across the life cycle, particularly for males. The levels of the enzyme are highest during the prepubertal years and after the age of 65, when sex hormones are at their lowest levels, which directly parallels the periods of highest prevalence for neuroleptic-induced PK (Robinson 1975; Robinson et al. 1972). Testosterone is known to be a more potent suppressor of monoamine oxidase activity than estrogen (Zeller and Davis 1980). For the younger males in our study, ages 10.3, 13.3, and 13.6, with atypical PK and without major affective symptomatology, we can thus speculate that the atypical PK manifestation may be contributed to by a particular biochemical vulnerability based on their prepubertal status, perhaps having to do with the activity of monoamine oxidase.

Recent reports of related work have very specifically defined biochemical gender differences in the expression of PK (Richardson et al. 1992, 1993). This work revealed a significant sex and platelet monoamine oxidase activity interaction in relation to both PK prevalence and severity in elderly psychiatric patients. Given that elderly patients and prepubertal children share the common factor of low levels of sex hormones, there may be more relevance to the child-elderly comparison than would be thought at first.

Aside from the issue of atypicality, we have highlighted three cases with severe symptom levels of PK. These findings are particularly surprising given that both patients B and G were receiving thioridazine, which has the highest anticholinergic potency of any of the other neuroleptics used in the 10 children. It is possible that we may be seeing an unexpected paradoxical reaction to the anticholinergic potency of this drug in these patients in reference to the severity of their PK. Further, patient B, a female with a diagnosis of major depression, showed both an atypical and a typical PK pharmacology and no TD symptoms. We can say that her particular vulnerability to symptom severity may be contributed to by her neurochemical status relating to the significant associations reported between affective symptoms and PK that we quoted earlier (Craig et al. 1985; Galdi 1983; Johnson 1981; Richardson et al. 1988). Patient G showed only PK symptoms and had only an atypical PK pharmacology. He was a prepubertal male, and we have discussed the vulnerability of that particular age and sex status.

The last case, patient E, was not being treated with thioridazine but with trifluoperazine at the evaluation when her PK scores were highest. She was 15.5 years old with a chart diagnosis of schizophreniform disorder. She showed coexisting TD and PK, substantial symptoms in both disorders, and typical pharmacology in both disorders. This patient had a family history of psychiatric hospitalization, which we have reported to be a significant risk factor for TD development (Richardson et al. 1991). She also had a behavioral history that included suicide attempts, stealing, and arson. It would have been helpful if we had performed a psychiatric status evaluation to determine whether she was experiencing any affective symptoms that would have demonstrated the affective symptoms/PK vulnerability association discussed.

The data that we have presented on our case studies allow us to feel confident in suggesting to clinicians that they be especially aware of the possibility of atypical and severe PK in prepubertal males and in patients of both sexes with affective components to their illness. In our previous work, we had found a high prevalence of PK in children and adolescents (at rates comparable to adults), the PK persisting beyond neuroleptic discontinuation, and a significant association between the development of PK and the length of the continuous neuroleptic treatment period prior to evaluation (Richardson et al. 1991). The cumulative effect of these data on PK establishes this disorder to be of prime concern in the use of neuroleptics in children and adolescents.

The atypicality in our TD symptoms was seen in two patients, one male and one female (patients D and F). For patient D, an adolescent male with a major affective disorder, the TD emerged after a decrease in anticholinergic exposure. There has been some limited work in adults that shows a heterogeneity in TD pharmacology in regards to anticholinergic activity in some patients (Casey and Denney 1977; Lieberman et al. 1988). There is, however, a body of work that indicates that, for most adult patients, anticholinergic treatment temporarily aggravates or uncovers TD symptoms (Baldessarini et al. 1980; Casey et al. 1981; Gardos et al. 1978; Gerlach 1979).

Patient F, an adolescent female with conduct disorder, had shown an atypical emergence of TD with a higher neuroleptic dose. Another report in a scant literature of treatment-emergent dyskinesias in adolescents has a related finding of atypicality (Polizos and Engelhardt 1978)—that is, of a positive correlation between dose and TD symptoms, but in the opposite direction. In that study, the only two children in a sample of child psychiatric patients with treatment-emergent dyskinesias showed an atypical reduction in symptoms with neuroleptic dose reduction. These findings can be considered to be related to the concept of initial dyskinesias, a little-known syndrome described as occurring primarily in younger patients (Casey et al. 1981; Gerlach

1985; Gerlach and Korsgaard 1981). The dyskinetic symptoms can be seen to increase or emerge after an increase in neuroleptic dosage and to decrease after a discontinuation of neuroleptic. It is considered to be an acute rather than a tardive phenomenon and may respond to treatment with antiparkinson agents. The two syndromes of initial dyskinesias and TD, however, are closely related, and the distinction may be of more academic than clinical relevance. Clinicians who treat children and adolescents, however, should be aware that dyskinesias that emerge with changes to higher doses of neuroleptics may well respond to treatment with antiparkinson agents.

We have previously defined risk factors for the development of TD in children and adolescents to be a family history of psychiatric hospitalization and a behavioral history that does not include assaultiveness (Richardson et al. 1991). We have further suggested that the very high rate of withdrawal-emergent dyskinesia in children and adolescents (seen much less frequently in adults), the low rate of treatment-emergent dyskinesia (seen at much lower rates than in adults), and the atypicality we and others have reported in the limited literature on treatment-emergent dyskinesias lead to the notion of differing neurochemical substrates in the dyskinesias in children and adolescents compared with those in adults (Campbell et al. 1983; Gualtieri et al. 1980; Richardson et al. 1991).

In conclusion, the data of this chapter highlight the responsibility of the field of child and adolescent psychopharmacology to establish a rubric that anticipates marked heterogeneity and an atypicality of treatment response from expected patterns at the very least in terms of neurological side effects. It further places on the clinicians serving these populations the responsibility to establish a schedule of rigorous and frequent monitoring for the neurological side effects of neuroleptics with no prior expectations and especially no complacencies.

References

Baldessarini RJ: Chemotherapy in Psychiatry, Revised Edition. Cambridge, MA, Harvard University Press, 1985

Baldessarini RJ, Cole JO, Davis JM, et al: Tardive Dyskinesia: A Task Force Report. Washington, DC, American Psychiatric Press, 1980

Campbell M, Grega DM, Green WH, et al: Review: neuroleptic-induced dyskinesias in children. Clin Neuropharmacol 6:207–222, 1983

Casey DE, Denney D: Pharmacological characterization of tardive dyskinesia. Psychopharmacology (Berlin) 54:1–8, 1977

Casey DE, Gerlach J, Korsgaard S: Clinical pharmacological approaches to evaluating tardive dyskinesia, in Clinical Pharmacology in Psychiatry: Neuroleptics and Antidepressant Research. Edited by Usdin E, Dahl S, Gram LF, et al. London, Macmillan, 1981, pp 369–382

Craig TJ, Richardson MA, Pass R, et al: Measurement of mood and affect among schizophrenic inpatients. Am J Psychiatry 142:1272–1277, 1985

Davis JM: Organic therapies, in Comprehensive Textbook of Psychiatry/IV, 4th Edition, Vol 2. Edited by Kaplan HI, Sadock BJ. Baltimore MD, Williams & Wilkins, 1985, pp 1481–1569

Galdi J: The causality of depression in schizophrenia. Br J Psychiatry 142:621–625, 1983

Gardos G, Cole JO, Tarsy D: Withdrawal syndromes associated with antipsychotic drugs. Am J Psychiatry 135:1321–1324, 1978

Gerlach J: Tardive dyskinesia. Dan Med Bull 26:209–245, 1979

Gerlach J: Pathophysiological mechanisms underlying tardive dyskinesia, in Dyskinesia: Research and Treatment. Edited by Casey DE, Chase TN, Christensen AV, et al. New York, Springer-Verlag, 1985, pp 98–103

Gerlach J, Korsgaard S: Classification and prevalence of neuroleptic-induced hyperkinetic movement disorder, in Biological Psychiatry. Edited by Perris C, Struwe G, Jansson B. Amsterdam, Elsevier, 1981, pp 844–851

Gualtieri CT, Barnhill J, McGimsey J, et al: Tardive dyskinesia and other movement disorders in children treated with psychotropic drugs. J Am Acad Child Adolesc Psychiatry 19:491–510, 1980

Johnson DAW: Studies of depressive symptoms in schizophrenia, I: the prevalence of depression and its possible causes. Br J Psychiatry 139:89–101, 1981

Lieberman J, Lesser M, Johns C, et al: Pharmacologic studies of tardive dyskinesia. J Clin Psychopharmacol 8 (suppl):57S–63S, 1988

Polizos P, Engelhardt DM: Dyskinetic phenomena in children treated with psychotropic medications. Psychopharmacol Bull 14:65–68, 1978

Richardson MA: Neuroleptic-Induced Parkinsonism: Current Concepts: Proceedings of New York State Office of Mental Health Second Annual Research Conference. Albany, NY, NYS Office of Mental Health, 1989, p 15

Richardson MA, Casey DE: Tardive dyskinesia status: stability or change. Psychopharmacol Bull 24:471–475, 1988

Richardson MA, Craig TJ: The coexistence of parkinsonism-like symptoms and tardive dyskinesia. Am J Psychiatry 139:341–343, 1982

Richardson MA, Pass R, Craig TJ, et al: Factors contributing to the prevalence and severity of tardive dyskinesia. Psychopharmacol Bull 20:33–38, 1984

Richardson MA, Pass R, Bregman Z, et al: Tardive dyskinesia and depressive symptoms in schizophrenics. Psychopharmacol Bull 21:130–135, 1985

Richardson MA, Pass R, Craig TJ: The coexistence of parkinsonism-like symptoms and tardive dyskinesia, in Biological Psychiatry, 1985: Developments in Psychiatry, Vol 7. Edited by Shagass C, Josiassen RC, Bridger WH, et al. New York, Elsevier Science Publishing, 1986a, pp 1211–1213

Richardson MA, Haugland G, Pass R, et al: The prevalence of tardive dyskinesia in a mentally retarded population. Psychopharmacol Bull 22:243–249, 1986b

Richardson MA, Pass R, Bregman Z: Contrasts between patients' characteristics associated with tardive dyskinesia vs those associated with parkinsonism-like symptoms, in Tardive Dyskinesia: Biological Mechanisms and Clinical Aspects. Edited by Wolf E. Washington DC, American Psychiatric Press, 1988, pp 109–122

Richardson MA, Casey DE, Bitter I: Elderly psychiatric patients: parkinsonism, sex, and MAO relationships. Biol Psychiatry (suppl) 25:73A, 1989a

Richardson MA, Suckow R, Whittaker R, et al: The plasma phenylalanine/large neutral amino acid ratio: a risk factor for tardive dyskinesia. Psychopharmacol Bull 25:47–51, 1989b

Richardson MA, Casey DE, Lin SP: Tardive dyskinesia five year outcome: a descriptive analysis. Paper presented at New Clinical Drug Evaluation Unit Conference, Alcohol, Drug Abuse and Mental Health Administration, US Department of Health and Human Services, Key Biscayne, FL, June 1989c

Richardson MA, Haugland G, Craig TJ: Neuroleptic use, parkinsonian symptoms, tardive dyskinesia, and associated factors in child and adolescent psychiatric patients. Am J Psychiatry 148:1322–1328, 1991

Richardson MA, Casey DE, Bitter I: Parkinson-like symptoms, MAO levels and Haldol levels in elderly psychiatric patients. Paper presented at Fifth International Amine Oxidase Meeting, Galway, Ireland, August 1992

Richardson MA, Read L, Reilly M, et al: Significant interactions: gender, parkinsonism, tardive dyskinesia and biochemical variables. Paper presented at Conference on Women and Minority Issues in Schizophrenia, Schizophrenia Branch, National Institute of Mental Health, Bethesda, MD, May 1993

Richelson E: Antimuscarinic and other receptor-blocking properties of antidepressants. Mayo Clin Proc 58:40–46, 1983

Richelson E: Neuroleptic affinities for human brain receptors and their use in predicting adverse effects. J Clin Psychiatry 45:331–336, 1984

Robinson DS: Changes in monoamine oxidase and monoamines with human development and aging. Federation Proceedings 34:103–107, 1975

Robinson DS, Nies A, Davis JN, et al: Ageing, monoamines, and monoamine oxidase levels. Lancet 1:290–291, 1972

Simpson GM, Angus JWS: Drug induced extra-pyramidal disorders. Acta Psychiatr Scand Suppl 46:1–58, 1970

Simpson GM, Lee JH, Zoubok B, et al: A rating scale for tardive dyskinesia. Psychopharmacology (Berlin) 64:171–179, 1979

Zeller EA, Davis JM: Protein content and monoamine oxidase activity in platelets. Schizophr Bull 6:267–274, 1980

CHAPTER 4

Haloperidol in Hospitalized Schizophrenic Children

Elizabeth Kay Spencer, M.D.
Vivian Kafantaris, M.D.
Maria V. Padron-Gayol, M.D.
Carl R. Rosenberg, Ph.D.

Although neuroleptic medication is well established as an effective treatment for acute and chronic schizophrenia in adulthood (Kane 1987), many questions remain unanswered about psychopharmacological treatment of schizophrenic children (Beitchman 1985; Campbell et al. 1991; McClellan and Werry 1992). This limited fund of information, despite rapid advances in the field of child psychopharmacology (Campbell and Spencer 1988), reflects several factors. First, despite an estimated lifetime prevalence of 1%, schizophrenia is rare before adolescence. Childhood-onset schizophrenia has been estimated to be 50 times rarer than is adult-onset schizophrenia (Karno and Norquist 1989).

Second, issues of diagnosis and classification complicate what knowledge can be gleaned from the literature and applied to current understanding of this disorder in children. The existence of children presenting with adultlike schizophrenic symptoms has been recognized since the turn of the century (DeSanctis 1906). Both Bleuler (1911/1950), using the diagnosis of dementia praecox, and Kraepelin (1919), who coined the term *schizophrenia,* reported that a small number of their adult patients had experienced childhood onset of their illness. The work of Bender (1947), among others, led to broadening of the concept of schizophrenia in childhood, with the result that the term *childhood schizophrenia* came to refer to psychotic children who now would be considered diagnostically heterogeneous. Rutter (1972) called attention to the use of "Childhood schizophrenia . . . as a generic term to include an astonishingly heterogeneous mixture of disorders with little in common other than their severity, chronicity, and occurrence in childhood" (p. 315). Thus review of the psychiatric literature preceding the publication of DSM-III (American Psychiatric Association 1980) requires thoughtful appraisal of the actual clinical presentation of patients diagnosed with "childhood schizophrenia." By current criteria, some would be diagnosed with infantile autism or psychotic disorder other than schizophrenia.

Finally, very little psychopharmacological research has been conducted in young schizophrenic patients diagnosed by modern criteria, either children or adolescents. Until two recent pharmacological studies, one at the Child Psychiatry Research Branch, National Institute of Mental Health (NIMH) (Gordon et al. 1994), and a second described in this chapter, there have been no double-blind, controlled neuroleptic studies in schizophrenic children.

A growing current literature about the diagnosis and phenomenology of childhood-onset schizophrenia, however, strengthens the foundation for pharmacological investigation in these young patients. Since publication of DSM-III in 1980, children and adolescents have been diagnosed schizophrenic by essentially the same criteria as those used for schizophrenic adults; minor changes reflecting developmental differences followed in DSM-III-R (American Psychiatric Association 1987). An increasing number of reports have documented that children can meet DSM-III or DSM-III-R criteria for schizophrenia and that schizophrenic children display the same clinical features as do adults.

A corollary assumption has been that psychotic symptoms in schizophrenic children may be ameliorated by the same medications that are effective in adults. This hypothesis has influenced clinical practice but, until recently, has not been tested in double-blind, controlled trials. In this chapter, we review current knowledge about the pharmacological treatment of childhood-onset schizophrenia and describe early results in a 10-week, double-blind, controlled study of the safety and efficacy of haloperidol in hospitalized prepubertal schizophrenic children, ages 5–12 years, diagnosed by DSM-III-R criteria. Initial findings in the first 14 subjects, previously reported for 12 subjects (Spencer et al. 1992), are discussed in the context of clinical and research issues relevant to neuroleptic treatment of this disorder in preadolescent children.

Background

The limited literature with bearing on pharmacological treatment of schizophrenic children includes four categories of papers, which together provide a foundation for further inquiry. First of interest are early pharmacological studies, the majority antedating DSM-III, which concern drug treatment of psychotic children. Within heterogeneous groups of patients are child and adolescent schizophrenic subjects treated with neuroleptic medication (for review, see Campbell 1985). Agents employed included haloperidol (LeVann 1969; Naruse et al. 1982), pimozide (Debray et al. 1972; Pangalila-Ratulangi 1973), and thiothixene (Simeon et al. 1974). Given the small patient numbers and a degree of retrospective uncertainty about diagnostic precision, results of these studies bear cautious interpretation; treatment benefits, however, were noted.

A second group of papers concerns pharmacological studies in schizophrenic adolescents. As with children, little research has been conducted, but data from three studies prior to 1990 are available (for review, see Campbell et al. 1991).

Pool et al. (1976) conducted the only double-blind, placebo-controlled neuroleptic trial in this age group, demonstrating the superiority of haloperidol and loxapine to placebo. The study involved 75 patients, ages 13–18 years, who had acute schizophrenia or chronic schizophrenia with acute exacerbation. The mean loxapine dose was 87.5 mg/day (612.5 mg/day chlorpromazine equivalents [CPZ-EQ]), with a range of 25–200 mg/day (175–1,400 mg/day CPZ-EQ); mean haloperidol dose was 9.8 mg/day (490 mg/day CPZ-EQ), with a range of 2–16 mg/day (100–800 mg/day

CPZ-EQ). Realmuto et al. (1984) compared thioridazine with thiothixene in 21 chronically ill adolescent schizophrenic patients, ages 11.75–18.75 years. They reported comparable efficacy and differing side-effect profiles for the two drugs, and that only about half the subjects on either agent improved. The mean thioridazine dose was 178 mg/day, with a range of 91–228 mg/day; mean thiothixene dose was 16.2 mg/day (405 mg/day CPZ-EQ), with a range of 4.8–42.6 mg/day (120–1,065 mg/day CPZ-EQ). Siefen and Remschmidt (1986) found that treatment with the atypical neuroleptic clozapine resulted in significant improvement for several patients with schizophrenia who either had failed to respond to or had experienced side effects on typical neuroleptics. Of 21 patients, including 12 who were younger than age 18 years, 11 were found to show marked improvement or remission of symptoms. The mean clozapine dose was 352 mg/day (704 mg/day CPZ-EQ), with a range of 254–700 mg/day (508–1,400 mg/day CPZ-EQ).

At the Child Psychiatry Branch, NIMH, where an ongoing, double-blind, controlled study of clozapine is in progress (Gordon et al. 1994), 11 adolescent patients (8 males and 3 females) with childhood-onset schizophrenia, diagnosed by DSM-III-R criteria, received clozapine in an open 6-week trial (Frazier et al. 1994). For study admission, these chronically ill patients were required to have had poor outcome with at least two previous neuroleptic trials, either because of persisting impairment or severe side effects. Receiving a mean clozapine dose of 370.5 mg/day (741 mg/day CPZ-EQ), with a range of 125–825 mg/day (250–1,650 mg/day CPZ-EQ), the group showed substantial overall improvement on several measures.

The third group of papers, focusing on diagnostic and phenomenological issues in young patients diagnosed schizophrenic by DSM-III or DSM-III-R criteria, refer to or discuss the use of neuroleptic medication. Although these papers do not present results of controlled pharmacological studies, they often pertain to the preadolescent age group and illustrate clinical experience with medicating schizophrenic children. As a group, these papers build on the work of Kolvin (1971), whose observations contributed to the establishment of infantile autism as a separate diagnostic entity in DSM-III. Kolvin differentiated infantile psychoses (before age 3 years) from late-onset childhood psychoses (5–15 years) according to clinical features now seen as corresponding to characteristic features of infantile autism and childhood-onset schizophrenia. He described the medication response of four patients with late-onset psychosis, all 11 years of age or older on acute onset of psychotic symptoms, who "at least initially, under cover of phenothiazine therapy, managed to return to school" (Kolvin 1971, p. 18). After an unspecified period of time, one patient was "functioning extremely well," one was "at least not deteriorating further," and the other two were "doing relatively poorly" (Kolvin 1971, p. 18).

In a retrospective study on the Bellevue Hospital Center Children's Inpatient Psychiatric Unit, Green et al. (1984) used DSM-III diagnostic criteria to compare 24 prepubertal schizophrenic and 25 autistic patients, with 24 children with conduct disorder as control subjects. The results of this study replicated Kolvin's (1971) finding that schizophrenia and infantile autism are distinct clinical entities. The schizophrenic children, differentiated from the autistic group by later onset of psychosis and other variables, were 15 males and 9 females, ages 6.7–11.11 years. A case vignette describes an 8-year-old schizophrenic boy whose overall neuroleptic treatment response was suboptimal. During his index episode at age 5, he appeared to benefit from chlorpromazine. On recurrence of psychotic symptoms when he was age 8, he failed to respond to thioridazine and was hospitalized, with fluctuating response to treatments, including haloperidol.

In a later article involving an expanded study sample of 38 children, Green et al. (1992) reported optimal dose ranges of neuroleptic medications received by 35 children, ages 5.7–11.11 years (mean age 9.6 years), some of whom received trials of more than one medication: chlorpromazine, 75–400 mg/day, for 12 subjects; trifluoperazine, 2–13 mg/day (60–390 mg/day CPZ-EQ), for 4 subjects; and haloperidol, 1–6 mg/day (50–300 mg/day CPZ-EQ), for 15 subjects. Overall, the children are described as relatively treatment resistant.

At the University of California at Los Angeles, where a number of investigators have studied childhood-onset schizophrenia, Russell et al. (1989) evaluated the phenomenology of childhood-onset schizophrenia in 35 subjects, 24 males and 11 females, ages 4–13 years (mean 9.54), who met DSM-III criteria. Ten subjects were receiving thioridazine and one was receiving chlorpromazine, with a mean dose of 143 mg/day, ranging from 50 to 375 mg/day. During administration of a newly developed semistructured interview, none of the 11 subjects on medication was noted to show clinical evidence of sedation.

Two studies from New Zealand also have referred to the use of neuroleptic medication for young schizophrenic patients. Kydd and Werry (1982) reported on 15 subjects, 8 males and 7 females, whose overall age range was 10–15 years; 9 were ages 13–15. By DSM-III criteria, 11 were diagnosed schizophrenic. Of the other 4, diagnosed with schizophreniform psychoses because of duration of illness less than 6 months, 3 were felt to be potentially schizophrenic. All 15 patients were treated with antipsychotic medication: 12 received thioridazine, 2 received fluphenazine decanoate, and 1 received trifluoperazine. As converted by the authors to CPZ-EQ, the mean maximum dose was approximately 400 mg/day (range, 75–900 mg/day), and the mean dose on discharge was approximately 200 mg/day (range, 75–500 mg). Acute positive symptoms, noted as hallucinations, delusions, and thought disorder, improved more than negative symptoms, such as withdrawal and blunted affect. With all the patients medicated, however, the effect of medication on outcome could not be fully assessed.

Using DSM-III-R criteria, Werry et al. (1991) later conducted a follow-up study of 59 psychotic child and adolescent patients. In the introductory remarks of this article, the authors define early-onset schizophrenia as beginning before age 18, with further separation into very-early-onset before age 13, as opposed to adolescent-onset schizophrenia from 13–17. Among several probable characteristics of very-early-onset patients, resistance to antipsychotic treatment is included but noted as requiring confirmation.

The mean age at onset of psychotic illness for the 59 patients was 13.9 years, with a range of 7–17 years; 10 had onset before age 13. The mean follow-up period was 5 years, with a range of 1–16 years. By initial diagnoses, 34 subjects were schizophrenic, 13 were schizophreniform, 9 had bipolar affective disorder, 1 was schizoaffective, and 2 had psychotic depression. Follow-up revealed increased proportions of bipolar disorder and schizoaffective disorder. On rediagnosis, 30 were schizophrenic, 23 were bipolar, and 6 were schizoaffective. Half of those found to be bipolar and 5 of 6 with schizoaffective disorder initially had been diagnosed schizophrenic. For all the schizophrenic group, rediagnosis confirmed the initial diagnosis; 90% were receiving neuroleptic medication. The authors emphasized the importance of longitudinal follow-up to minimize the risk of misdiagnosis and consequent use of inappropriate medication.

The fourth paper category relevant to psychopharmacological research in schizophrenic children is represented by case reports. These address neuroleptic treatment of patients with childhood-onset schizophrenia. One patient, a 13.5-year-old boy with onset of symptoms 2 years prior to hospitalization, was treated with haloperidol, receiving up to 40 mg/day (2,000 mg/day CPZ-EQ) and with optimal response at 30 mg/day (1,500 mg/day CPZ-EQ) (Meyers et al. 1980). His serum haloperidol levels suggested a faster rate of neuroleptic metabolism than that seen in adults.

Another patient, an 8.5-year-old boy, initially was thought to have attention-deficit/hyperactivity disorder and as an outpatient received a course of methylphenidate (Perlmutter et al. 1989). He required hospitalization for behavioral deterioration and worsening psychotic symptoms and subsequently was rediagnosed as schizophrenic. Over a period of several months, he received trials of three neuroleptics: thioridazine, up to 150 mg/day (150 mg/day CPZ-EQ); haloperidol, up to 6 mg/day (300 mg/day CPZ-EQ); and molindone, up to 75 mg/day (750 mg/day CPZ-EQ). His optimal therapeutic response was achieved on molindone, 50 mg/day (500 mg/day CPZ-EQ). Several subsequent case reports also have described children and adolescents with schizophrenia who have benefited from treatment with clozapine (Birmaher et al. 1992; Jacobsen et al. 1994; Mozes et al. 1994; Towbin et al. 1994).

A Study of Haloperidol Treatment of Hospitalized Schizophrenic Children

The goals of the study reported on in this chapter are to evaluate, under double-blind, placebo-controlled conditions, the safety and efficacy of haloperidol in the treatment of hospitalized children, ages 5–12 years, who have been diagnosed schizophrenic by

DSM-III-R criteria. This research was conducted on the Bellevue Hospital Center Children's Inpatient Psychiatric Unit. This 15-bed unit, for children ages 2–11 years, is the New York City acute care child inpatient psychiatric facility for a catchment area comprising most of the borough of Manhattan.

This study follows a long history of child psychopharmacological research on the unit. Numerous treatment studies, including several using haloperidol, have been conducted in two other patient populations: young autistic children (Anderson et al. 1984; Campbell et al. 1978, 1982, 1988) and explosively aggressive children with conduct disorder (Campbell et al. 1984; Platt et al. 1984). Prior experience with schizophrenic children on this unit also culminated in the clinical studies cited above: the initial report comparing schizophrenic, autistic, and conduct-disordered children (Green et al. 1984) and later reports concerning phenomenology (Green and Padron-Gayol 1986; Green et al. 1992). The double-blind, placebo-controlled haloperidol study was initiated on the unit in 1989. Treatment results for the first 14 subjects are described in this chapter. Data from this pharmacological study also have been reported in a preliminary report (Spencer et al. 1992) and elsewhere (Campbell et al. 1991; Spencer and Campbell 1994; Spencer et al. 1994).

The choice of haloperidol for the study reported on in this chapter was predicated first on the unit's previous research and clinical experience with haloperidol for the treatment of autistic children and aggressive children with conduct disorder. These studies demonstrated the efficacy and safety of haloperidol in those two child psychiatric populations. Second, the side-effect profile of haloperidol, as a less-sedating, high-potency neuroleptic, was judged to be preferable for young children, whose capacity to participate fully in school and age-appropriate activities potentially could be adversely affected by sedation.

Subjects

The subjects in this study were actively psychotic prepubertal boys and girls, 5–12 years of age, diagnosed as schizophrenic by DSM-III-R criteria. Their presenting psychiatric and behavioral symptoms, such as hallucinations, delusions, disordered thinking, suicidal or homicidal ideation, and impaired judgment, necessitated inpatient stabilization and treatment. Study subjects included children referred to the unit for hospitalization both from the Bellevue Hospital Center catchment area and through active recruitment in the metropolitan New York City area. Informed consent for study enrollment was obtained from parents or guardians, in accordance with regulations of the New York University Medical Center Institutional Board of Research Associates, the Bellevue Hospital Center, and the New York City Health and Hospitals Corporation.

Exclusion criteria for this study reflected efforts to conform precisely with DSM-III-R criteria, to minimize medical risk, and to attain a homogeneous clinical sample. Exclusion criteria were diagnoses of infantile autism, major affective illness (unipolar or bipolar), or mental retardation (unless psychological testing revealed deterioration from a previously documented level of function or indicated impingement of psychosis on higher potential); systemic disease; history of seizure disorder; tardive or withdrawal dyskinesia; and receipt of psychoactive medication within 4 weeks of beginning double-blind treatment. Children receiving medication on admission to the unit were withdrawn from medication for 2 weeks before entering placebo baseline.

Design

The study was 10 weeks in duration and employed a crossover design. After an initial 2-week placebo baseline period, children diagnosed as schizophrenic by concurrence of three child psychiatrists and showing target psychotic symptoms of severity warranting a medication trial proceeded to 8 weeks of double-blind treatment. By random assignment, each child received either haloperidol for 4 weeks, followed by placebo for 4 weeks, or, alternatively, placebo for 4 weeks, followed by haloperidol for 4 weeks.

During placebo baseline, the study subjects, like all children admitted to the unit, underwent comprehensive assessment by the clinical ward staff, including child psychiatrists, psychologists, nurses, social workers, and activity therapists, as well as classroom teachers in the special education department of New York City Public School No. 106, which is adjacent to the unit. General pediatric consultation, as needed, and pediatric neurology consultation with electroencephalogram were obtained. Laboratory assessment included admission blood tests and a pretreatment electrocardiogram, repeated at the end of each treatment period. During placebo baseline, the children concurrently were evaluated by the research team. A battery of standardized rating scales, detailed later, was completed twice. Diagnostic assessment included the Diagnostic Interview for Children and Adolescents—Revised (Reich and Welner 1990).

During each 4-week, double-blind treatment, dosage was regulated individually, with adjustment according to clinical response and emergence of adverse effects. The dose range was 0.5–10.0 mg/day (25–500 mg/day CPZ-EQ), in three divided doses given at 8 A.M., 12 noon, and 3 P.M. Starting dose was 0.5 mg/day (25 mg/day CPZ-EQ). During the first 2 weeks of the treatment period, dosage was increased approximately every 3 days, by increments of 0.25–0.5 mg (12.5–25 mg CPZ-EQ). Optimal therapeutic dose was determined by clinical assessment as the dose at which the child showed maximal improvement in target symptoms in the absence of, or with minimal, side effects. Optimum dose then was maintained for the duration of the 4-week period.

Treatment response was assessed by a battery of rating scales, among which were several developed by the NIMH Psychopharmacology Research Branch (Guy 1976; *Psychopharmacology Bulletin* 1985). The battery was completed four times, twice during placebo baseline and again at the end of each double-blind treatment. Ratings were conducted by several raters, all blind to treatment status, whose observation of the child occurred in a variety of settings. The research team of three child psychiatrists, after an interview with the child, completed the Children's Psychiatric Rating Scale (CPRS) and Clinical Global Impressions (CGI) (Guy 1976; *Psychopharmacology Bulletin* 1985), the Brief Psychiatric Rating Scale for Children (BPRS-C) (Gale et al. 1986), the Abnormal Involuntary Movements Scale (*Psychopharmacology Bulletin* 1985), and the Simpson Abbreviated Dyskinesia Rating Scale (Simpson et al. 1979). Three additional scales were completed by the classroom teacher, the unit head nurse, and research nurse, respectively: the Conners Teacher Questionnaire, the Conners Parent-Teacher Questionnaire, and the Nurse's Global Impressions (Guy 1976; *Psychopharmacology Bulletin* 1985).

At the end of the study, before the child's double-blind treatment code was broken, the unit clinical and research staff met together to discuss the child's progress. The staff attained a Global Clinical Judgments consensus rating (as adapted from Campbell et al. 1984). This rating compared the child's response during each of the two double-blind treatments to baseline. The child first was rated unchanged, improved, or worsened; then, the degree of change was rated mild, moderate, or marked.

Data for 12 of the children were analyzed using a 2 × 2 crossover analysis of variance, testing for carryover and period effects as well as treatment effects (Spencer et al. 1992). One-tailed *P* values were reported, with the rationale that the target symptoms were unlikely to worsen on haloperidol.

Results

The 14 subjects presented in this chapter, including 12 described previously (Spencer et al. 1992), were 10 boys and 4 girls who were ages 5.5–11.75 years (mean, 8.89 years) on admission to the study. All 14 patients presented with auditory hallucinations and delusions. Nine of 14 experienced visual hallucinations. The content of the children's hallucinations and delusions was often related, involving perceptual phenomena attributed to, as well as beliefs about, such entities as a demon, a witch, a baby, a rat, a movie projector, and characters from cartoons and horror movies. Thought disorder and inappropriate affect each were observed in 12 subjects.

All 14 children improved on haloperidol, and after the study they continued to receive haloperidol. Their mean optimal haloperidol dose during double-blind administration was 1.95 mg/day (97.5 mg/day CPZ-EQ). The optimal dose range was 0.5–3.5 mg/day (25–175 mg/day CPZ-EQ) or 0.02–0.12 mg/kg/day (1–6 mg/kg/day CPZ-EQ). For 9 of 14, the optimal haloperidol dose was 0.04–0.06 mg/kg/day (2–3 mg/kg/day CPZ-EQ). Of three subjects requiring higher doses for optimal response, the two whose optimal doses were highest were sisters, receiving 3.0 and 3.5 mg/day (150 and 175 mg/day CPZ-EQ).

By Global Clinical Judgments consensus ratings, comparing each treatment response to baseline, all 14 patients improved on haloperidol; the degree of improvement was marked in 10, moderate in 3, and mild in 1. On placebo there was mild improvement, with two exceptions: one subject showed moderate improvement, and one worsened from baseline.

During haloperidol administration, side effects in these 14 subjects were transient, resolving either with dose maintenance or reduction. The two most common side effects were drowsiness, noted in 10, and drooling, noted in 4. Less common were dizziness, masklike facies, and tongue discomfort, each of which were observed in 2 subjects. Mild upper extremity cogwheel rigidity, decreased arm-swing while walking, mild ticlike lip movements, and minimal vermicular tongue movements each occurred in one subject. A total of four acute dystonic reactions in 3 subjects resolved with a single oral dose of diphenhydramine elixir 25 mg, followed by reduction of the study medication dose.

As reported previously, the following preliminary analyses of CPRS, CGI, BPRS-C, and the Global Clinical Judgments consensus rating data—conducted for 12 of these 14 subjects—support the clinical observation that they showed greater improvement on haloperidol than on placebo (Spencer et al. 1992). For this group of 12, analyses showed no carryover or period effects. Significant haloperidol treatment effects were found for several items, including the Global Clinical Judgments consensus ratings ($P = .0025$). On the CGI (Table 4–1), both items for "severity of illness" and "global improvement" showed significant haloperidol treatment effects, as did the BPRS-C "total pathology" scores ($P = .003$). On the CPRS (Table 4–2), four of eight selected items pertinent to schizophrenia also were significant: "ideas of reference," "persecutory" (which by the CPRS definition includes persecutory delusions), "other thinking disorders," and "halluci-

Table 4–1. Haloperidol treatment effect: Clinical Global Impressions ratings in 12 schizophrenic children

Item	Baseline	Placebo	Haloperidol	One-tailed *P*
1. Severity of illness	5.15	4.33	2.99	.0007
2. Global improvement	3.58	2.58	1.54	.02

Source. Spencer et al. 1992.

Table 4–2. Haloperidol treatment effect: mean Children's Psychiatric Rating Scale ratings in 12 schizophrenic children

Item	Baseline	Placebo	Halo-peridol	One-tailed *P*
57. Ideas of reference	2.09	2.03	1.31	.04
58. Persecutory	3.06	2.68	1.31	.01
59. Other thinking disorders	3.48	2.89	2.11	.04
61. Hallucinations	4.25	3.46	1.97	.04
17. Suspicious affect	2.33	1.68	1.25	.16
19. Blunted affect	2.37	2.76	2.26	.08
60. Delusions	4.16	3.33	2.61	.07
62. Peculiar fantasies	3.44	2.73	2.56	.13

Source. Spencer et al. 1992.

nations." The item for "delusions" (those other than persecutory) did not attain significance.

Discussion

Data from the study are the first to be published from a double-blind, placebo-controlled study of neuroleptic response in prepubertal schizophrenic children diagnosed by modern criteria; thus comparison data from other recent pharmacological studies are lacking. Like the other studies reviewed earlier in this chapter, this study has identified a group of prepubertal children who demonstrate the same schizophrenic symptomatology shown by adults. Early findings from this study suggest that schizophrenic children may respond to lower doses than those noted in the literature, which have been based on clinical experience rather than on the results of prospective pharmacological studies. The mean optimal haloperidol dose for the first 14 subjects in this study was 1.95 mg/day (97.5 mg/day CPZ-EQ), with a range of 0.5–3.5 mg/day (25–175 mg/day CPZ-EQ). In CPZ-EQ, these doses are lower than or overlap those in the phenomenological papers and the two case reports previously cited.

All of the first 14 hospitalized schizophrenic children in this 10-week, double-blind study improved on haloperidol and, because of the degree of their improvement, continued receiving haloperidol after completing the study protocol. The clinical observation that the children showed greater improvement on haloperidol than on placebo is supported by several preliminary analyses of rating data. During this 10-week study, in which haloperidol was administered for 4 of the 8 double-blind treatment weeks, haloperidol side effects were transient and resolved either with dose maintenance or following dose reduction. The initial results of this study thus appear to indicate that haloperidol is both efficacious and safe for short-term treatment of hospitalized schizophrenic children.

As a group, in the context of this inpatient study, the first 14 children were treatment responsive, rather than treatment resistant. The clinical benefit of haloperidol appears to exceed that attributable to placebo effect or to the effect of hospitalization alone. Beyond this short-term study of haloperidol in schizophrenic children, future goals will be to evaluate whether neuroleptic treatment remains a safe and efficacious component of their care.

References

American Psychiatric Association: Diagnostic and Statistical Manual of Mental Disorders, 3rd Edition. Washington, DC, American Psychiatric Association, 1980

American Psychiatric Association: Diagnostic and Statistical Manual of Mental Disorders, 3rd Edition, Revised. Washington, DC, American Psychiatric Association, 1987

Anderson LT, Campbell M, Grega DM, et al: Haloperidol in the treatment of infantile autism: effects on learning and behavioral symptoms. Am J Psychiatry 141:1195–1202, 1984

Beitchman JH: Childhood schizophrenia: a review and comparison with adult-onset schizophrenia. Psychiatr Clin North Am 8:793–814, 1985

Bender L: Childhood schizophrenia. Am J Orthopsychiatry 17:40–56, 1947

Birmaher B, Baker R, Kapur S, et al: Clozapine for the treatment of adolescents with schizophrenia. J Am Acad Child Adolesc Psychiatry 31:160–164, 1992

Bleuler E: Dementia Praecox or the Group of the Schizophrenias (1911). Translated by Zinkin J. New York, International Universities Press, 1950

Campbell M: Schizophrenic disorders and pervasive developmental disorders/infantile autism, in Diagnosis and Psychopharmacology of Childhood and Adolescent Disorders. Edited by Wiener JM. New York, Wiley, 1985, pp 113–150

Campbell M, Spencer EK: Psychopharmacology in child and adolescent psychiatry: a review of the past five years (review article). J Am Acad Child Adolesc Psychiatry 27:269–279, 1988

Campbell M, Anderson LT, Meier M, et al: A comparison of haloperidol, behavior therapy and their interaction in autistic children. Journal of the American Academy of Child Psychiatry 17:640–655, 1978

Campbell M, Anderson LT, Cohen IL, et al: Haloperidol in autistic children: effects on learning, behavior, and abnormal involuntary movements. Psychopharmacol Bull 18:110–112, 1982

Campbell M, Small AM, Green WH, et al: Behavioral efficacy of haloperidol and lithium carbonate: a comparison in hospitalized aggressive children with conduct disorder. Arch Gen Psychiatry 41:650–656, 1984

Campbell M, Adams P, Perry R, et al: Tardive and withdrawal dyskinesia in autistic children: a prospective study. Psychopharmacol Bull 24:251–255, 1988

Campbell M, Spencer EK, Kowalik SC, et al: Schizophrenic and psychotic disorders in childhood and adolescence, in Comprehensive Textbook of Child and Adolescent Psychiatry. Edited by Wiener JM. Washington, DC, American Psychiatric Press, 1991, pp 223–239

Debray P, Messerschmitt P, Lonchamp D, et al: L'utilisation du pimozide en pedopsychiatrie (the use of pimozide in child psychiatry). La Nouvelle Presse Medicale 1:2917–2918, 1972

DeSanctis S: On some varieties of dementia praecox, in Revista Speriomentale de Freniatria e Medicina Legale della Alienazioni Mentale. New York, Brunner/Mazel, 1906, pp 141–165

Frazier JA, Gordon CT, McKenna K, et al: An open trial of clozapine in 11 adolescents with childhood-onset schizophrenia. J Am Acad Child Adolesc Psychiatry 33:658–663, 1994

Gale J, Pfefferbaum B, Suhr MA, et al: The Brief Psychiatric Rating Scale for Children: a reliability study. Journal of Clinical Child Psychology 15:341–345, 1986

Gordon CT, Frazier JA, McKenna K, et al: Childhood-onset schizophrenia: an NIMH study in progress. Schizophr Bull 20:697–712, 1994

Green WH, Padron-Gayol M: Schizophrenic disorder in childhood: its relationship to DSM-III criteria, in Biological Psychiatry. Edited by Shagass C, Josiassen RC, Bridger WH, et al. New York, Elsevier, 1986, pp 1484–1486

Green WH, Campbell M, Hardesty AS, et al: A comparison of schizophrenic and autistic children. J Am Acad Child Adolesc Psychiatry 23:399–409, 1984

Green WH, Padron-Gayol M, Hardesty AS, et al: Schizophrenia with childhood onset: a phenomenological study of 38 cases. J Am Acad Child Adolesc Psychiatry 31:968–976, 1992

Guy W: ECDEU Assessment Manual for Psychopharmacology (DHEW Publ No ADM-76-338). Rockville, MD, 1976

Jacobsen LK, Walker M, Edwards JE, et al: Clozapine in the treatment of a young adolescent with schizophrenia. J Am Acad Child Adolesc Psychiatry 33:645–650, 1994

Kane J: Treatment of schizophrenia. Schizophr Bull 13:133–156, 1987

Karno M, Norquist GS: Schizophrenia: epidemiology, in Comprehensive Textbook of Psychiatry/V, 5th Edition, Vol 1. Edited by Kaplan HI, Sadock BJ. Baltimore, MD, Williams & Wilkins, 1989, pp 699–704

Kolvin I: Psychoses in childhood—a comparative study, in Infantile Autism: Concepts, Characteristics and Treatment. Edited by Rutter M. London, Churchill Livingstone, 1971, pp 7–26

Kraepelin E: Dementia Praecox and Paraphrenia. Translated by Barclay RM (from the 8th German Edition of the Textbook of Psychiatry). Edinburgh, Livingstone, 1919

Kydd RR, Werry JS: Schizophrenia in children under 16 years. J Autism Dev Disord 12:343–357, 1982

LeVann LJ: Haloperidol in the treatment of behavioural disorders in children and adolescents. Canadian Psychiatric Association Journal 14:217–220, 1969

McClellan JM, Werry JS: Schizophrenia. Psychiatr Clin North Am 15:131–148, 1992

Meyers B, Tune LE, Coyle JT: Clinical response and serum neuroleptic levels in childhood schizophrenia. Am J Psychiatry 137:483–484, 1980

Mozes T, Toren P, Chernauzan N, et al: Clozapine treatment in very early onset schizophrenia. J Am Acad Child Adolesc Psychiatry 33:65–70, 1994

Naruse H, Nagahata M, Nakane Y, et al: A multi-center double-blind trial of pimozide (Orap), haloperidol and placebo in children with behavioral disorders, using a crossover design. Acta Paedopsychiatrica 48:173–184, 1982

Pangalila-Ratulangi EA: Pilot evaluation of Orap (pimozide R6238) in child psychiatry. Psychiatria Neurologia Neurochirurgia 76:17–27, 1973

Perlmutter IR, Greenhill LL, Chambers W, et al: Grand rounds: childhood schizophrenia: theoretical and treatment issues. J Am Acad Child Adolesc Psychiatry 28:956–962, 1989

Platt J, Campbell M, Green WH, et al: Cognitive effects of lithium carbonate and haloperidol in treatment-resistant aggressive children. Arch Gen Psychiatry 41:657–662, 1984

Pool D, Bloom W, Mielke DH, et al: A controlled evaluation of loxitane in seventy-five adolescent schizophrenic patients. Current Therapeutic Research 19:99–104, 1976

Psychopharmacology Bulletin: Rating scales and assessment instruments for use in pediatric psychopharmacology research (special feature). Psychopharmacol Bull 21:765–770, 1985

Realmuto GM, Erickson WD, Yellin AM, et al: Clinical comparison of thiothixene and thioridazine in schizophrenic adolescents. Am J Psychiatry 141:440–442, 1984

Reich W, Welner Z: Diagnostic Interview for Children and Adolescents—Revised. St Louis, MO, Washington University Press, 1990

Russell AT, Bott L, Sammons C: The phenomenology of schizophrenia occurring in childhood. J Am Acad Child Adolesc Psychiatry 28:399–407, 1989

Rutter M: Childhood schizophrenia reconsidered. Journal of Autism and Childhood Schizophrenia 2:315–337, 1972

Siefen G, Remschmidt H: Behandlungsergebnisse mit clozapin bei schizophrenen jugendlichen (Clozapine in the treatment of adolescents with schizophrenia). Z Kinder Jugendpsychiatr 14:245–257, 1986

Simeon J, Saletu B, Saletu M, et al: Thiothixene in childhood psychoses. Adv Biochem Psychopharmacol 9:519–534, 1974

Simpson GM, Lee JH, Zoubok B, et al: A rating scale for tardive dyskinesia. Psychopharmacology (Berlin) 64:171–179, 1979

Spencer EK, Kafantaris V, Padron-Gayol M, et al: Haloperidol in schizophrenic children: early findings from a study in progress. Psychopharmacol Bull 28:183–186, 1992

Spencer EK, Campbell M: Children with schizophrenia: diagnosis, phenomenology, and pharmacology. Schizophr Bull 20:713–725, 1994

Spencer EK, Alpert M, Pouget ER: Scales for the assessment of neuroleptic response in schizophrenic children: specific measures derived from the CPRS. Psychopharmacol Bull 30:199–202, 1994

Towbin KE, Dykens EM, Pugliese RG: Clozapine for early developmental delays with childhood-onset schizophrenia: protocol and 15-month outcome. J Am Acad Child Adolesc Psychiatry 33:651–657, 1994

Werry JS, McClellan JM, Chard L: Childhood and adolescent schizophrenic, bipolar and schizoaffective disorders: a clinical and outcome study. J Am Acad Child Adolesc Psychiatry 30:457–465, 1991

CHAPTER 5

Cognitive Effects of Neuroleptic Treatment in Children With Conduct Disorder

Laurence L. Greenhill, M.D.
Jeffrey M. Halperin, Ph.D.
Joseph Barmack, Ph.D.

Neuroleptic medication has been used to treat a variety of behavior disorders in school-age children, such as conduct disorder and attention-deficit/hyperactivity disorder (ADHD) (Gittelman-Klein et al. 1976; Greenhill et al. 1981, 1985; Werry and Aman 1975). Evidence suggests that these medications can reduce the severe symptoms of aggressivity and hyperactivity. A review by Whitaker and Rao (1992) listed four controlled studies (Barker and Fraser 1968; M. Campbell et al. 1982a, 1982b, 1984; Wong and Cock 1971) involving 122 child and adolescent patients with aggressive behavior problems who were treated with neuroleptics. These studies showed that haloperidol, chlorpromazine, and lithium were all effective in the reduction of aggressive behaviors.

Indications for the use of neuroleptics in children and adolescents as found in the *Physicians' Desk Reference* (Medical Economics 1991) are not diagnostically specific but rather, as in the case of thioridazine,

> for the treatment of severe behavioral problems in children marked by combativeness and/or explosive hyperexcitable behavior (out of proportion to immediate provocations), and in the short-term treatment of hyperactive children who show excessive motor activity with accompanying conduct disorders consisting of some or all of the following symptoms: impulsivity, difficulty sustaining attention, aggressivity, mood lability, and poor frustration tolerance. (p. 1951)

Although neuroleptics enjoyed considerable popularity in child and adolescent inpatient services in former years (Lipman et al. 1978), the long-term risks for tardive dyskinesia (Gualtieri et al. 1980) and neuroleptic malignant syndrome (Teicher and Glod 1990) have been major reasons that clinicians have been reluctant to prescribe them routinely.

Children who receive psychopharmacological treatments often present with behavioral difficulties accompanied by academic impairment. Yet, as pointed out by Platt et al. (1984), neuroleptic treatment studies involving children and adolescents have not always reported outcome measures that assess behavioral and cognitive components. Sedation, a common side effect of neuroleptics at all ages, and particularly at the neuroleptic dosages commonly used to quell aggressiveness in children, may interfere with the sustained attention necessary for learning in the classroom. Similar effects, known as "fog states," have been reported in children and adolescents taking neuroleptics to reduce the tics and coprolalia associated with Tourette's syndrome. Although two studies (Klein 1991; Wong and Cock 1971) reported that neuroleptics did not impair cognitive functioning at doses that reduced behavioral symptoms, other studies (Cunningham et al. 1968; Helper et al. 1963; Platt et al. 1984; Sprague et al. 1970) reported that behaviorally effective doses of neuroleptics produce performance decrements on certain laboratory tasks. Various explanations have been suggested to explain these discrepant findings, including differences in diagnoses, symptom severity, dosages, time of administration, duration of treatment, and the outcome measures used to assess cognitive performance (Klein 1991; Platt et al. 1984).

Measuring Cognitive Effects of Neuroleptics

The need for collecting cognitive performance measures when treating children and adolescents with psychopharmacological agents has been well established. Children, unlike adult psychiatric patients, may not complain about their behavioral and psychological difficulties. As a result, outcome measures frequently depend on the observations of parents, teachers, and clinicians who may or may not directly observe the child in routine but quite uncontrolled situations. Cognitive measures, on the other hand, can be carried out in a highly controlled manner in a laboratory and have been used to test the magnitude of drug effects objectively in more clearly defined domains. These tasks investigate whether centrally acting medications have effects on cognitive processing, in addition to modifying the child's emotional response to social situations. Therefore, through the use of cognitive measures, one can determine whether medications that slow or minimize aggressivity and hyperactivity also modify information processing, memory, recall, and speech. These effects could be quite detrimental if children who are already academically impaired have their classroom performance further reduced.

Because psychostimulant treatments involving methylphenidate or dextroamphetamine produce strong effects on a wide variety of noninvasive laboratory measures at predictable times after dosing with the medication, a wide variety of tasks have been devised and replicated across studies. Positive effects of stimulant treatment have been reported on short-term memory tasks involving recognition of simple but unfamiliar pictures on cards in the Paired Associates Task (Kupietz 1991; Sprague and Sleator 1977); tests of impulsivity and cognitive style, such as the Matching Familiar Figures Task (Kagan 1966); and tests that determine the child's ability to plan, such as the Porteus Maze test (Porteus 1959). Other performance tasks lend themselves to automation, with microcomputers running the cognitive tasks and collecting the patient responses.

Experimenter-paced tasks involving simple but rapidly repeated signals have been widely used to validate clinical findings in pediatric psychopharmacology. In one study (Sprague and Sleator 1977), the Paired Associates Task showed an optimal effect at a lower dose of methylphenidate (0.3 mg/kg), whereas the same children had a better behavioral response at a higher dose (1.0 mg/kg). This study has important implications; it suggested that there might be a dissociation between cognitive and social effects of a medication. Concern over such a possibility may be responsible for the tradition of setting methylphenidate dosages by weight, a trend that developed since the study was published, despite the evidence for there being no relation between oral dosage, patient weight, plasma level, or behavioral response (Rapport et al. 1989).

Effects of Neuroleptics on Cognitive Performance

It is widely held by clinicians that neuroleptics, so useful in ameliorating thought disorder in schizophrenic adults, cause cognitive impairment in children. Early research (M. Campbell et al. 1971) suggested that aliphatic phenothiazines produced sedation and depressed performance on laboratory tasks. In an uncontrolled study, McAndrew et al. (1972) reported that three children, treated with thioridazine (40–200 mg/day), failed to show the expected progress over 1 year on the Stanford Achievement Test. Goldstone and Lhamon (1976) reported that haloperidol reduced the rate of temporal auditory information processing in adult patients with Tourette's disorder and schizophrenia who did not differ from control volunteers until placed on neuroleptics. Sprague et al. (1980), working with mentally retarded adolescents (Full Scale Wechsler Intelligence Scale for Children—Revised [WISC-R] IQ 30–50), found a discrepancy between doses that led to social cooperativeness (high doses) and those that optimized learning on a color identification task (low doses).

A number of factors have proven critical in determining the cognitive performance of children while on neuroleptics. Dose of medication, as shown earlier, can be critical, as well as the time of day that the dose is administered. Severely disturbed inpatients with undersocialized conduct disorder had impaired performance on the Porteus Maze task when their haloperidol medication was administered throughout the day instead of at bedtime

(Platt et al. 1984). Klein (1991) agreed, stating that the sedating effects of these medications occurs early in absorption and thus could be reduced in the daytime if the medications are given only at bedtime.

Quality of performance on these laboratory measures is affected by the type of task, whether it is experimenter paced or subject paced, and by the social environment, whether the test takes place in a classroom or a laboratory. Winsberg and Yepes (1978) found that the sedation seen in the laboratory is lessened in the more stimulating environment of the classroom. The duration of the treatment study also has a bearing on the cognitive test performance. If the tests are repeated weekly over a period of months, the resulting "practice effects" often improve the child's performance. These factors compromise the generalizability of results from laboratory-based cognitive tasks.

Continuous Performance Test

The Continuous Performance Test (CPT) is an experimenter-paced vigilance task widely used in psychiatric research. The test involves memory, sustained attention, and inhibition of impulsive responses. For these reasons, it is suitable for detecting detrimental effects of neuroleptics on cognition. The test has excellent face validity for studying disorders of distractibility and inattentiveness in children because it indicates failures to detect target signals, analogous to ignoring or failing to follow a teacher in a classroom (Bergman et al. 1991).

The CPT also is a reliable method for objectively assessing inhibitory control (Sykes et al. 1973) relatively independent of other cognitive processing abilities (Halperin et al. 1991a, 1991b, 1991c) and uncontaminated by motor effects (Aman 1978). First employed to study changes in brain-damaged adults objectively (Rosvold et al. 1956), it has been used extensively with a wider range of clinical populations, including schizophrenia (Nuechterlein 1983), learning disabilities, personality disorders, ADHD (Halperin et al. 1991a, 1991b, 1991c, 1992; Klorman et al. 1984; Rapoport et al. 1980; Sykes et al. 1971, 1972, 1973), and conduct disorder (Klee and Garfinkel 1983), and with children at risk for schizophrenia (Erlenmeyer-Kimling and Cornblatt 1978; Rutschman et al. 1977). The CPT is also sensitive to amphetamine drug effects in both ADHD and control children (Rapoport et al. 1978). All of these populations, at baseline and before treatment, have shown impaired CPT performance compared with control subjects.

The CPT has good test-retest reliability over periods of several months (Halperin et al. 1991a), and several lines of data support its construct validity for assessing attention and impulse control (Halperin et al. 1988, 1991a, 1991b, 1991c). CPT performance is uncontaminated by motor effects (Aman 1978) and is independent of activity level. Kornetsky et al. (1959) stated that poor CPT performance indicates a low state of central arousal. This allows competing internal and external stimuli to interfere with complete registration of the target. Mackworth (1981) theorized that only when the subject sustains an attentional test-taking set to the relevant stimuli can the subject perform well. Conners (1994) suggested that drug-induced decreases in the commission error rate may be dependent on drug inhibition of cortical hyperarousal. The CPT is reported to be able to measure inhibitory control (Sykes et al. 1973), to be sensitive to amphetamine drug effects in both ADHD and control children (Rapoport et al. 1978), and to show differences between control children and those in high-risk populations (Erlenmeyer-Kimling and Cornblatt 1978).

The classic CPT measure is a "fixed" or "static" experimenter-paced task. Thus the rate of stimulus presentations is under the control of the examiner, not the subject. Sitting still, watching the CPT monitor, remembering instructions, and tolerating the dull repetition of stimuli all contribute to the frustration, boredom, and stress experienced by an ADHD child taking the test. Even so, this laboratory measure may not present the full stress such a child might experience in a classroom of 30 children. Whalen et al. (1979) found that a teacher-paced task can elicit more inattention and disruptiveness than self-paced tasks.

The CPT measures sustained attention by requiring the subject to detect infrequently appearing "target" letters or "signals" interspersed among many "nontargets," all presented rapidly on a screen. Most CPTs depend on visual detection, although auditory CPT formats have been explored for assessing attention during positron-emission tomography studies (Zametkin et al. 1990). Some describe the procedure as a "watch" or "vigil" comparable to sitting at a sonar or radar screen, attempting to detect enemy ships or planes that might emerge at any time from a background of "noise" or nonsignals (Bergman et al. 1991; Swets and Kristofferson 1970). The subject generally indicates the detection of a target signal by pressing a button or lifting a finger from a switch. Lapses in attention, when the subject fails to identify a target as it flashes on the screen, are scored as errors of omission (EOMs), or misses. Button presses to nontarget stimuli are scored as errors of commission (EOCs) or false alarms. These are shown diagrammatically in Figure 5–1.

Although the CPT is oftentimes discussed as a single task, the nature of the stimuli, rates of presentation, and response demands vary considerably. Some investigations select a single target, such as the letter *X* (Klorman et al. 1984). Others require that a fixed two-letter sequence appear, such as an *A* followed by an *X* (the CPT AX task) (Sykes et al. 1973), whereas others require a more flexible sequential target such as the same stimulus occurring two times in a row. It is likely that these procedural differences result in partially distinct processes being assessed by the different CPTs.

In addition, more complicated CPTs have been used. Cornblatt and colleagues employ a "playing card" CPT with younger children (Bergman et al. 1991) that uses pictures of playing cards, including the 2–10 of clubs and the 2–10 of spades. Subjects are asked to respond whenever they are shown two cards in a row that are exactly the same (e.g., the 8 of clubs followed by the 8 of clubs). The authors pointed out that this is more difficult than the standard CPT AX task because the patient must store each num-

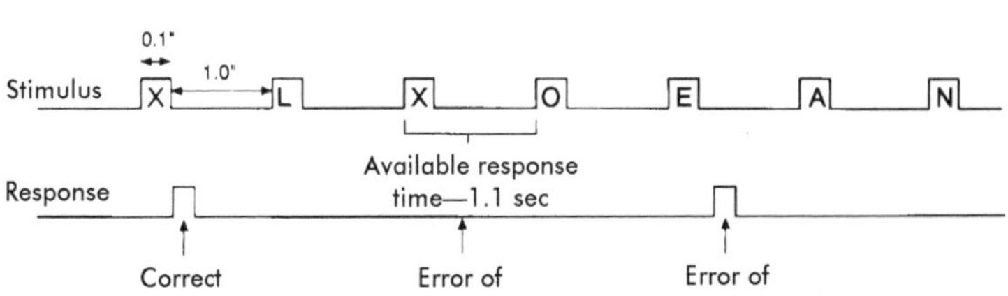

Figure 5–1. Diagram of the Continuous Performance Test indicating the timing of correct responses, errors of omission, and errors of commission in relation to the stimulus.

ber–playing card symbol stimulus in memory and attempt to match it with the next one.

Analysis of CPT data produces a variety of outcome variables. The hit rate is the number of correct detections divided by the total number of targets. Of greater interest in the analysis are the errors in performance. EOMs are assumed to reflect attentional dysfunction, particularly an inability to sustain attention, whereas EOCs may be associated with impulsivity. Halperin et al. (1991a, 1991b, 1991c) explained that the EOC can occur when the time necessary for full cognitive processing (necessary for identifying the stimulus and making an accurate response) is compromised for the sake of speed. An associated measure, the false alarm rate, is obtained by dividing the number of incorrect responses (EOCs) by the total of noncritical *A*s plus *X*s minus the number of targets. Several investigators have reported very high rates of EOCs in child psychiatric populations. Typical output data from experimenter-paced or static CPT studies in child psychiatry populations are listed below in Table 5–1.

Halperin's (1988, 1991a, 1991c) investigations suggest that EOCs may not measure a unitary construct. Rather, responses to different nontarget stimulus sequences within a CPT AX paradigm reflect distinct underlying processes. Not only do distinct subtypes of EOCs occur with different reaction times, but they are differentially related to teacher ratings of inattention and impulsivity. Halperin's group found that the *A*-not-*X* error occurred at fast reaction times and was associated with ratings of impulsivity and conduct problems. On the other hand, a response to an *X* not preceded by an *A* (X-only error) occurred at slow reaction times and, along with EOMs, was associated with teacher ratings of poor attention. Halperin found that A-only and random errors (response to a sequence containing neither an *A* or an *X*) are not associated with a unique reaction time pattern or ratings of any specific behavioral construct.

The Dynamic CPT

The CPT has been programmed to run on Apple and IBM-PC compatible computers (Klee and Garfinkel 1983). It also is commercially available on dedicated machines. There are many versions, varying in presentation rate, interstimulus interval (ISI), type of

Table 5–1. Continuous Performance Test fixed mode: age and performance data

Investigators	*N*	Age	Number of targets	Hit rate X mode	Hit rate AX mode	Analysis type
Crosby 1972	24	15	160X/120AX	96.1	92.7	Standard
Crosby 1972	24	9	160X/120AX	68.7	63.5	Standard
Rosvold et al. 1956	26	9	160X/120AX	82.6	79.4	Standard
Sykes et al. 1971	19	8	90AX in 600	82.3	77.4	Standard
Sykes et al. 1973	20	8.3	90AX in 600	—	62.0	Standard
Herman et al. 1977	10	7	—	86.9	—	Standard
J. Barmack, unpublished manuscript, March 1985	10	15.4	—	86.9	—	Standard
Rutschman et al. 1977	150	15.5	80 in 323	NA	NA	Signal detection
Cornblatt et al. 1988	30	7–12	—	—	—	Signal detection
Halperin et al. 1991a, 1991b, or 1991c	54	7–12	40 in 400	—	79.5	Standard
Halperin et al. 1991a, 1991b, or 1991c	138	7–11	40 in 400	—	91.5	Standard
Overall means, ages 7–15	—	—	—	80.1	70.6	

targets, and the presence or absence of distracter conditions. The most crucial aspect of a CPT is whether the CPT delivery of stimuli is independent of subject response. The original CPT was experimenter paced or "static" and used with adults. Although this type of control works well across different adult populations, it presents a distinct problem for studies in children. There is a developmental course to the ability to respond to the static CPT (Levy 1980). A version that challenges a 7-year-old will be easy for a 10-year-old. To combat this "ceiling" effect (Bergman et al. 1991), investigators have modified the CPT paradigm by degrading the quality of the image on the computer monitor, adding distracting voices in earphones, or making the target stimulus more complex.

One method of countering developmental effects is to adjust the rate of presentation—the ISI—based on the accuracy of the subject's identification of targets. This dynamic CPT has been used in the study of inpatients (Klee and Garfinkel 1983), nondisordered boys (Rapoport et al. 1980), and college students (Buchsbaum and Sostek 1980). By this technique, the rate of stimulus display is adjusted according to the quality of the subject's performance (i.e., the machine's pace is increased with a correct response) and is decreased when an error occurs. The primary measure of interest in a dynamic CPT is the ISI that a subject titrates to. Data from a number of studies utilizing the dynamic CPT are listed in Table 5–2.

Although the ISI duration appears to be shorter for subjects in the studies by Buchsbaum and Rapoport than those by J. Barmack's ("Attentional Tests in Child Psychiatric Populations," unpublished manuscript, March 1985), the ratio of critical to noncritical targets used in the former studies is very low (i.e., 10%, 5%, and 5%), whereas in Barmack's work a ratio between 18% and 29% was used. There are insufficient data points to draw conclusions about relationships between age and percentage of targets detected. However, the percentage of targets detected (hit rate) for the dynamic mode is well below those shown in Table 5–1 for the fixed mode. The performance of Barmack's control subjects (as measured by their EOCs, EOMs, and hits) compares favorably with the performances reported by Buchsbaum and Rapoport, except for the ISI. Note that the EOCs for the AX dynamic task were highest in the inpatient adolescent group. High EOCs and elevated ISI among inpatients suggest that the dynamic mode of

Table 5–2. Continuous Performance Test dynamic mode: age and performance data

Investigators	*N*	Age	Number of targets	Hit rate	Errors of commission	Errors of omission	Interstimulus interval (msec)
Buchsbaum and Sostek 1980	375	18	60 in 600	77	14.7	13.6	34.1
Rapoport et al. 1980	31	22.3	32 in 800	84	4.0	5.0	31.1
Rapoport et al. 1978	14	10.9	32 in 800	76	7.5	7.5	40.4
J. Barmack, unpublished manuscript, March 1985							
AX (inpatients)	8	15.3	120 in 516	78	32.0	26.4	56.3
X (inpatients)	8	15.3	120 in 408	—	21.4	16.4	60.1
Control subjects	9	15–40	100 in 556	78	11.7	13.3	43.6
Overall means	—	—	—	77.4	13.7	12.8	34.1

the CPT may be useful for evaluating medication effects in neuroleptic-treated children because the baseline rate of performance errors is very high, meaning that ceiling effects are unlikely to occur.

However, there are other problems with the dynamic CPT. The meaning of hits, misses, false alarms, and reaction time measures varies as a function of the ISI. Therefore, if subjects titrate to different ISIs, they cannot be compared on the other CPT variables. Second, the test slows down, and ISI increases for subjects who make more errors. Therefore, the total target test time increases. If the subject has a "sustained attention" deficit, the additional duration of the test should make the subject's performance even worse. Third, an implicit assumption of the dynamic CPT is that increasing the ISI makes the task easier whereas decreasing the ISI makes it harder. However, when Sykes et al. (1971, 1972, 1973) used a 1.5- and 1.0-second ISI, they found that the hyperactive children did worse with the longer ISI. This finding suggests that the condition was more difficult for them. If varying the ISI has differential effects across groups (or drug conditions), it confounds any comparisons that you may want to make. Fourth, accurate performance on a dynamic CPT can reduce the ISI to the point where the subject can no longer respond quickly enough to indicate detection before the next stimulus is presented. As a result, the number of errors will be artificially inflated. Depending on how the CPT handles the type of error, it can be extremely problematic. For example, if the ISI goes down to 400 milliseconds, and the subject responds with a reaction time of 650 milliseconds, the subject's response may not occur until after the next stimulus is presented. Does the subject's response get scored as two errors—a miss for the target stimulus and a false alarm for the next stimulus? This scenario could also play out with an intended incorrect response. At short ISIs, it will be difficult to determine to which stimulus the subject intended to respond.

Signal Detection and the CPT

Nuechterlein (1983) suggested that signal detection theory may be useful for analyzing CPT data. The conventional method of scoring CPT variables (EOM, EOC) does not allow for the separation of basic perceptual and attentional processes from motivational factors that might affect the subject's compliance with responding in a given manner. Using signal detection theory, Swets and Kristofferson (1970) found that the ability to detect the signal from nontargets, or perceptual sensitivity (d′), can be distinguished from motivational factors in response biases. This latter factor, or "log beta," is the attitude toward responding, which is characterized along a continuum from "conservative" (responding only to those signals when absolutely certain) to "lax" (responding to every stimulus).

Sensitivity refers to the distance between a hypothetical Gaussian noise distribution and the signal necessary for the subject to respond to it. Older boys and nondisordered children have higher d′ than do ADHD children, and amphetamine significantly increases d′ in younger ADHD children. The unit of sensitivity, d′, assumes normal variance in the noise and in the subject's responses and is most stable if the subject can report how certain he or she is when responding. The estimated sensitivity based on signal detection theory, P(A), does not require these assumptions and is a better fit with our population of school-age children with conduct disorders. P(A) could measure drug-related changes in sensitivity or attentiveness. This variable ranges between 0.5 (pure chance) and 1.0 (top accuracy). Neuroleptics, if they depress cognition, will depress P(A) during active drug treatment.

Parasuraman (1979) pointed out that perceptual sensitivity itself can fall off if the events being processed occur rapidly or if the target discrimination loads memory. Inattention, which is detected by an increase in error rate over time, can be a result of a failure to detect targets or, as Swets and Kristofferson (1970) pointed out, a change in decision criterion where the subject decides to become more conservative in calling a questionable signal a target. Because the CPT requires the maintenance of performance over time (van der Meere and Sergeant 1987), errors that occur often can be viewed as a deterioration in vigilance. Error rates increase as the CPT runs, with more errors occurring later in the task. The capacity to sustain attention deteriorates over time in lengthy monitoring tasks, but deterioration in performance may be confounded with changes in response criteria.

The other variable, log beta, generally measures attitudes to responding. In children with disruptive behavior disorders, log beta is high, meaning that they display a lax criterion to responding. Rapoport et al. (1978) reported that children with disruptive behavior disorders pushed the response button very often, even when the machine was off. If neuroleptics reduce impulsivity, the log beta should drop during treatment.

CPT Detection of Medication Effects

The CPT has been used in a number of psychopharmacology studies. All data have been collected in the laboratory, and most deal with acute medication effects rather than changes seen after months on a drug. No dose-response learning curves have been available, although two different doses of a drug have been compared in some studies. Tolerance and state-dependent learning effects have not been reported in these articles.

Neuroleptics have not shown consistent effects on laboratory-based cognitive tests, and the CPT is no exception. Wong and Cock (1971) found that low-dose haloperidol did not interfere with cognitive tests for 6 months. Werry and Aman (1975) studied both high (0.05 mg/kg/day) and low (0.025 mg/kg/day) fixed haloperidol doses administered for a 3-week period, which had different effects on CPT performance. The low dose facilitated performance on the CPT, whereas the high dose caused an impairment on a task of short-term memory. Platt et al. (1984) used higher haloperidol doses (0.096 mg/kg/day; range, 0.04–0.21) in 61 inpatients and tested before and after 4 weeks of drug treatment. Haloperidol caused a significant decrease in performance on the Porteus Maze test and a slowing of reaction time on a simple reaction time task. Klein (1991) treated 36 outpatient children (ages 6–12 years) diagnosed as ADHD with thioridazine (193 mg; range, 25–300 mg) for 4 weeks in a controlled study, comparing their performance with 41 children treated with placebo, and found little deterioration in performance on the CPT.

A Controlled Study of the Cognitive Effects of Molindone and Thioridazine

The CPT was used to assess the cognitive effects of neuroleptics on children during a controlled study of molindone hydrochloride. This medication had been proven effective, with improvement rates ranging from 25% to 50%. Anecdotal reports suggested molindone had positive effects in chronic schizophrenia, anxiety disorders, and depression, as reported in a review of 19 published studies involving 554 patients (Claghorn 1985). Twelve of these studies were double-blind and controlled. Four of six controlled studies of 200 schizophrenic adults showed that clinical improvement was maintained for 13 months or more at doses as high as 225 mg/day. Even so, the literature on this medication involves small trials, and there is a paucity of placebo-controlled designs. Most studies compare molindone to other neuroleptics (Hollister 1968; Kellner et al. 1976).

Two uncontrolled pediatric studies of molindone (M. Campbell et al. 1971; Renshaw 1977) have suggested that this medication might be well tolerated by children. One involved administration of molindone, 1–5 mg/day, to 10 preschool children with a broad range of diagnoses for a mean duration of 8 weeks (M. Campbell et al. 1971). Moderate improvement in clinical state was reported, with four or five children showing a reduction in irritability, hyperactivity, and impulsivity. Seven of these children showed a combination of stimulant and sedative effects; six children developed extrapyramidal signs, including tremor, restlessness, gross body movements, and acute dystonia. Renshaw (1977) conducted another open trial in 22 child patients between the ages of 5 and 12 years with diverse psychiatric diagnoses. She found that doses of 10–15 mg/day of molindone produced significant improvements on the Children's Psychiatric Rating Scale (CPRS) after 11–42 days of treatment. The psychotic children improved more rapidly than the nonpsychotic children. Roughly one-third of her patients developed treatment-emergent symptoms, including drowsiness (eight patients), nausea (four patients), and skin changes (four patients). Six patients had to stop molindone prematurely.

Additionally, an 8-week, double-blind molindone study was conducted by Greenhill et al. (1985). In this chapter, we report on the CPT findings from that study to assess cognitive "cost" for treatment with these neuroleptics.

Method

Sample. Subjects eligible for inclusion in the study were children between the ages of 6 and 11 who were inpatients on the

Children's Psychiatric Research Unit of the New York State Psychiatric Institute with a diagnosis of undersocialized conduct disorder with aggressivity. Two child psychiatrists, using a diagnostic checklist based on the DSM-III (American Psychiatric Association 1980) definition, were required to arrive at this diagnosis independently. Signs of conduct disorder had to be evident for a minimum duration of 6 months cross-situationally and include a history of aggressive behavior resulting in damage to objects or persons and some evidence, on history or interview, of poor interpersonal relationships with peers. Hospitalization took place on a 12-bed pediatric psychiatry ward for children between the ages of 5 and 14 years. Once admitted to the ward, the children had to obtain a score of greater than 4 on the CPRS for the following items: angry affect, suspiciousness, fighting with peers, and temper outbursts (Guy 1976), and they had to remain above these scores over the first 2 weeks on the ward. The protocol also required a score of 1.8 or greater on Trites et al. (1982) factor 1 (hyperactivity) of the Conners Teacher Questionnaire (CTQ) and a score of greater than 25 on the Inpatient Aggression Scale (IAS), an instrument developed for this study.

Exclusion criteria included a prior history of neuroleptic treatment, certain medical disorders (anemia, liver disease), endocrine disease (diabetes, precocious puberty), neurological disease (seizure disorders, multiple sclerosis or tumor), or treatment with medications that could alter prolactin measures (prednisone, anticonvulsants, dextroamphetamine) within the past month. Of the 46 children initially eligible, 15 were excluded from randomization into active treatments when their CPRS scores fell below 4 prior to drug treatment. The remaining 31 subjects were randomly assigned to one of the active drug treatment groups (molindone or thioridazine).

The characteristics of the two study groups are shown in Table 5–3. As can be seen, there was only one female. The mean ages of the two groups were not significantly different (molindone, 9.8 years; thioridazine, 10.3 years). Six were white, 14 were black, and 11 were Hispanic, but the ethnic distribution did not differ significantly between the two drug groups nor did the mean social class rating (4.3 for the molindone group and 4.25 for the thioridazine group). Mean full-scale WISC-R IQ differed significantly in the two groups ($t = 4.55$, $P < .01$), with the molindone group

Table 5–3. Demographic data: inpatient school-age children with conduct disorder (mean ± SD)

Variable	Molindone (N = 15)	Thioridazine (N = 16)
Age at start	9.8 ± 1.7	10.3 ± 1.8
WISC-R FS IQ*	81.9 ± 15.6	71.5 ± 12.0
Socioeconomic status		
Two factor	55.5 ± 14.7	56.3 ± 14.3
Social class	4.3 ± 1.1	4.25 ± 1.0
Ethnicity (Caucasian/ Hispanic/black)	2/6/7	4/5/7
Sex ratio (M:F)	15:0	15:1

Note. WISC-R FS = Wechsler Intelligence Scale for Children—Revised, full scale.
*$P < .01$.

showing a higher mean score (81.9) than the thioridazine group (71.5). However, the rate of school failure did not differ significantly by chi-square analysis.

Preadmission behaviors were collected by interviewing parents and teachers. Histories of repeated tantrums, frequent fights with adults and peers, and truancy occurred in a majority of the children, with no significant difference between the two drug groups. The frequencies of runaway and fire-setting behaviors also did not differ significantly between the two groups. Social histories revealed evidence of parental neglect, physical abuse, chronic asthma, and foster care, distributed equally between the two treatment groups.

The 31 children maintained their aggressive behavior during the first week, the off-drug period, and the second week, the single-blind, placebo period, and continued to exceed the study's threshold scores. More than 80% displayed physical aggression toward objects and peers, verbal aggression, noncompliance with rules, and behaviors that disrupted group activities at a frequency of three or more times per week. Thus, their aggressivity and noncompliant behaviors were transsituational and created serious management and limit-setting problems on the ward, as they had previously done at home and at school.

Study design. After parents or guardians signed a statement of informed consent, the 31 children participated in an 8-week, double-blind, parallel-design drug study, diagrammed in Figure 5–2. Children spent the first week in the hospital off drug to observe the effects of hospitalization and then were switched to placebo for a second week to determine if they still met criteria for study (phase P1). Children had the option of moving through the off-drug and placebo (P1) phases within 48 hours if they scored 35 or greater on the IAS and scored 4 or more on each of three aggressive items on the CPRS (Guy 1976), including items 11, 48, and 50. This occurred rarely, with one child from each treatment condition being moved back on medication 5 days into the final placebo period.

Random assignment was made to either thioridazine (16 children) or molindone (15 children) at the end of the first placebo phase (P1). Starting with week 3, all children entered into a double-blind, fixed-flexible dosing schedule on active neuroleptic, either thioridazine or molindone. At the beginning of this dose-ranging period, drug intake was arbitrarily begun at 5 "active tab-

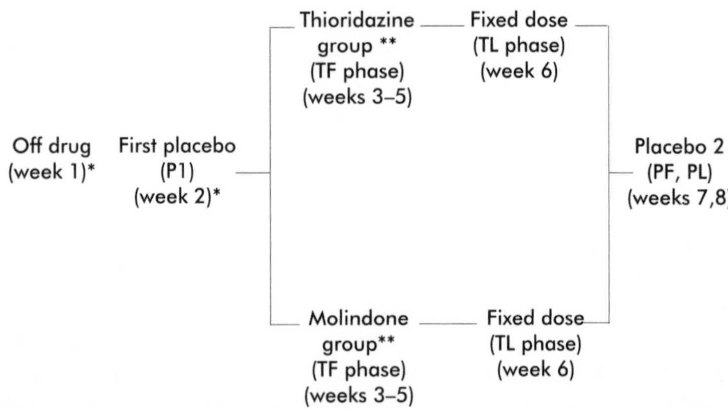

Figure 5–2. Molindone pediatric study: flowchart (inpatient, A-B-A design). *Placebo phases can be shortened to 48 hours if aggression is severe. **Active drug can be thioridazine (2.5–10 mg/kg/day) or molindone (0.5–2.0 mg/kg/day). Randomization occurs at end of week 2.

lets," equivalent to 125 mg of thioridazine or 25 mg of molindone, based on our pilot study (Greenhill et al. 1981). For the next 3 weeks, their drug dose was varied by the clinician based on the IAS scored by the nurses. The final week on active drug, week 6, was designated phase TF (final treatment week), and all subjects were returned to the five active tablets. All outcome measures were performed during this final week on fixed dosage. The study concluded with a repeat placebo period, which consisted of 2 weeks, week 7 (phase PF for final placebo) and week 8 (phase PL, for last placebo). This lengthy placebo period was utilized to compensate for thioridazine carryover effects. At the end of the study, all children were discharged on thioridazine.

Outbursts of aggression were treated with time-outs and seclusion. No additional medications were used for prn purposes. Anticipated neuroleptic side effects were treated, including the use of benztropine for acute dystonia and antacids for any epigastric discomfort.

Behavior ratings. Dependent measures were gathered weekly and included three scales administered by nurses: the 10-item Conners Abbreviated Parent-Teacher Questionnaire, the items common to both the Conners Parent Rating Scale and the Conners Teacher Rating Scale (Guy 1976); the Dosage Order Treatment Emergent Symptoms Scale (DOTES) (Guy 1976); and the IAS, based on items 1–11 of the CPRS (Guy 1976). The IAS recorded type of aggression (verbal or physical), the target of aggressive acts (physical objects, peers, or adult staff), and their frequency. Reliability studies on this new scale were carried out, with two of the nurses showing a high reliability on tests of 10 inpatients not enrolled in the study ($r = .82, P < .05$). Routine tests for liver abnormalities, complete blood count, and slit-lamp examinations for lenticular opacities were carried out before and after the study. Weekly weight changes were also assessed. At study termination, nurses filled out a Clinical Global Impressions rating scale (Guy 1976) to evaluate overall improvement seen in each child during the 8 weeks of treatment.

CPT procedures. Subjects were individually tested in a single room located in a quiet part of the inpatient service. The test apparatus consisted of a dedicated portable computer, which was capable of administering two different types of CPT tasks: the static CPT and a dynamic CPT. The computer controlled a light-emitting diode display, 3 by 2 inches. Each subject took a 20-minute CPT once per week, at the same time and day, for the duration of the 8-week study period. This CPT battery consisted of one 8-minute static CPT run followed by one dynamic CPT run, which varied in length (depending on performance) from 8 to 10 minutes.

For the static CPT, the computer set the signal stimulus (an *X* sequence) for a duration of 0.8 seconds and an ISI of 130 milliseconds; 11 other letters were also shown as nontargets. Every time a target appeared, the subjects were supposed to lift their finger from highly sensitive microswitches situated below their dominant hands.

The machine was then switched into the dynamic mode. Subjects were run using the same test time of 8 minutes. Target letter sequences (*A* followed by *X*) were termed hot trials, whereas other combinations were considered nontarget sequences or cold. A total of 800 letters were presented, which contained 32 *AX* combinations (4%). The sequences also contained 96 *A*s and 96 *X*s (each 12%).

During the dynamic mode, the microcomputer began the task at an initial setting of stimulus duration of 150 milliseconds and an ISI of 1 second. As the child performed the task, the CPT's microcomputer reviewed the accuracy of response after every five target stimuli. Because control subjects usually make less than 5% errors, the error rate was increased by reducing the ISI by 5% following correct identifications. Conversely, the ISI was increased by 5% following EOCs or EOMs. If the sum of the late (correct) responses plus EOCs equaled zero, the speed of presentation was increased by 1/16 of the current ISI. The other values—including the stimulus duration, the available response time, and the upper ISI limit—were proportionally adjusted. If the late (correct) response plus EOCs equaled 2, no change in rate was made. If the sum was greater than 2, the rate was slowed. The net effect is for the machine to seek a rate at which the patient responds 60% correct and 40% late. Because the object was to achieve the shortest interval between signals, subjects were told to operate at their fastest rate of accurate signal processing. The ISI, therefore, was one of the main dependent measures in this dynamic CPT task.

Statistical analyses. Summary scores included the hit rate, EOMs (misses), false alarm rates, and ISI for the last 400 stimuli. Because distributions of all measures were skewed, all data analyses were done on log-transformed numbers. Conditional probabilities for hits and false alarms were obtained: both the index of discriminability (P[A]) between hot and cold trials and a weighted measure of the hits relative to the false alarms (log beta) were computed. Calculation of P(A) is done by transforming the empirically derived hit rate (HR) and false alarm rate (FAR) (assumed to be normally distributed) into Z scores: using the method of Buchsbaum and Sostek (1980), the P(A) is defined as the Z(HR) – Z(FAR) and log beta is calculated as a ratio of the standardized ordinate of the individual's hit rate and false alarm rate – Y(HR)/Y(FAR).

Behavioral ratings were obtained from physicians, nurses, and ward teachers, using the CTQ and the CPRS. Data reduction and the repeated-measures design and analysis are described elsewhere (Greenhill et al. 1985). Data analysis utilized multiple *t* tests with independent samples, analysis of variance in a repeated-measures design, and chi-square tests; Bonferroni corrections (Miller 1981) of alpha were made to protect against Type 1 errors. All *P* values are expressed in a two-tailed probability format.

Results

Behavior ratings. The inpatient baseline (off-drug) behavior of the two groups did not differ significantly. Using the Trites et al. (1982) norms for the CTQ, both groups exceeded the 1.8 threshold score for ADHD. Mean CTQ scores were 1.85 for the thioridazine group and 2.19 for the molindone group. Mean conduct scores on the CTQ were also high—1.65 for the thioridazine group and 1.5 for the molindone group. Both groups exceeded our threshold aggression summary score criterion (25) at the end of the first placebo period (P1): 27.1 for the thioridazine group and 29.0 for the molindone group. The mean severity scores on the baseline Clinical Global Impressions were 5.6 for the thioridazine group and 5.3 for the molindone group, falling between the "markedly ill" and "severely ill" categories. No significant differences were found for a large variety of demographic variables or Wide Range Achievement Test subscores on multiple *t*-test comparisons.

Drug doses and side effects. At the beginning of the dose-ranging period, drug intake was arbitrarily begun at 5 active tablets, which yielded a total daily dose of 125 mg of thioridazine (125 mg chlorpromazine equivalents [CPZ-EQ]) or 25 mg of molindone (250 mg CPZ-EQ). During the initial dose-ranging part of the protocol, 9 molindone-treated children (60%) required a dosage adjustment: 4 required decreases and 5 increases. The remaining 4 children stayed at the starting level of 25 mg/day. Of the thioridazine subjects, 13 (81%) required further dosage adjustment: 5 decreasing and 8 increasing dosages. For the 3 weeks of fixed dosing, the mean thioridazine dose was 214.1 ± 122.1 mg/day (4.64 mg/kg/day), which is equivalent to the same dose of chlorpromazine. The mean molindone dose was 29.3 ± 11.1 mg/day (0.8 ± 0.25 mg/kg/day), which is equivalent to 293 mg/day of chlorpromazine.

The thioridazine group began with a mean weight of 40.4 ± 8.4 kg (range, 29–60.3 kg) and finished with a mean weight of 43.6 ± 10.0 kg (range, 29.2–66.5 kg). The molindone group began with a mean weight of 36.9 ± 7.6 kg (range, 25.4–48.3 kg) and finished with a mean weight of 38.2 ± 7.7 kg (range, 26.2–52.6 kg). These weight changes were not significant.

The mean thioridazine dosage rose from 134.3 mg/day to 214.1 ± 122.1 mg/day by the end of the flexible-dosing period. The mg/kg/day dose was to 5.1 ± 3.4 for the fixed-dosing period (week 4). The mean molindone dosage started at 23.4 mg (234 mg CPZ-EQ) but rose to 29.3 ± 10.9 mg/day (293 mg CPZ-EQ) by the end of the flexible-dosing period. However, during the fixed-dosing period, the weight-adjusted molindone dose was 0.78 ± 0.25 mg/kg/day.

A number of standard neuroleptic side effects were tracked by the nursing staff using the DOTES. These side effects were expressed as the mean percentage of the sample affected over the 4 weeks of active treatment and were corrected by subtracting the rate of similar complaints during the first placebo period. When these values were analyzed by week and by drug, no significant differences were found between the two treatments. There was a tendency for molindone to produce a higher rate of dystonic reactions than thioridazine and more often to require a change of dose because of toxicity. On the other hand, thioridazine-treated children had greater weight gain and slightly higher (but not significantly different) rates of sedation, dizziness, gastric upset, headache, and poorer compliance.

Behavior changes: placebo and active. Study rating form data were subjected first to a within-groups analysis, as shown in Table 5–4. Thioridazine and molindone produced significant symptom improvement compared with both pre- and posttreatment placebo periods. The thioridazine group showed significant changes from the first placebo period to the last week of active treatment, with significant decreases in CPRS ($P < .028$) and IAS ($P < .032$). In both cases, there were no significant differences in mean score between first and second placebo periods, and the IAS showed a significant increase ($P < .049$) at the final placebo period (2 weeks after the thioridazine was discontinued) over the last treatment week. The CPRS showed significant thioridazine-related improvements on the hostility, antisocial, and violence subscales when placebo periods were compared with various points in active treatment.

The molindone group also demonstrated within-group changes over the time of the study. CTQ scores fell significantly when both the first and last treatment weeks were compared with the first placebo period and showed a trend that was marginally significant over baseline scores after drug discontinuation ($P < .051$). The IAS showed significant improvement during the drug period when contrasted to both the first and second placebo periods. The CPRS revealed significant improvement on hostility, antisocial, and violence subscales for comparisons of placebo periods against the first or last week of treatment.

Between-groups analysis utilized an analysis of variance and covariance with repeated measures, as shown in Table 5–5. These procedures demonstrated that treatment effects were primarily time related. When the analysis was examined for drug × time interactions (including all changes in the comparisons of placebo week 1, treatment week 1, treatment week 4, and placebo week 2), any differential advantages for either drug treatment disappeared. Significant effects between drugs on the IAS were due to

Table 5–4. Within-group analysis by week: treatment-placebo comparisons (T values)

	Molindone (*N* = 15)		Thioridazine (*N* = 16)	
Rating scale	**Score**	***P***	**Score**	***P***
Conners 10-item scale				
P1 X TF	2.3	<.037	15.8	<.028
P1 X TL	2.4	<.035	15.8	<.028
TL X PF	—		—	
Inpatient Aggression Scale				
P1 X TF	3.6	<.003	—	
P1 X TL	2.6	<.023	2.4	<.032
TL X PF	2.2	<.053	2.2	<.049
CPRS hostile				
P1 X TF	—		4.3	<.001
P1 X TL	—		2.4	<.031
TL X PF	2.3	<.042	—	
CPRS antisocial				
P1 X TF	—		3.7	<.002
P1 X TL	3.4	<.012	—	
TL X PF	2.7	<.019	—	
CPRS violence				
P1 X TF	—		4.8	<.001
P1 X TL	2.7	<.018	3.3	<.005
TL X PF	3.1	<.01	3.2	<.007

Note. Data entered only if results were significant. P1 = first placebo week. TF = first treatment week. TL = last treatment week. PF = first week of second placebo period. CPRS = Children's Psychiatric Rating Scale.

time ($P < .001$); when the time × drug effects interaction was studied, any differences between the two drugs became nonsignificant ($F = 0.94$, $P < .4$). This was also true for the CPRS; the significant advantage for molindone ($F = 3.51$, $P < .019$) disappeared ($F = 0.94$, $P < .718$) when the drug × time interaction was computed. Thus, molindone and thioridazine both demonstrated significant improvement over baseline, and they also showed similar improvement over time.

Table 5–5. Analysis of variance and covariance using repeated measures of F scores comparing drugs across groups over time

Rating measure	Time effect	Drug × time
Inpatient Aggression Scale	6.05***	0.94
Conners 10-Item Scale	3.51*	0.45
CPRS aggression	4.52**	0.75
CTQ hyperactivity	0.3	1.32
CTQ conduct disorder	0.4	1.53
CPRS hostility	6.71***	0.47
CPRS antisocial	5.51***	0.66
CPRS hyperactivity	2.74*	1.38
Weight gain	22.91***	3.54[a]

Note. CTQ = Connors Teacher Questionnaire. CPRS = Children's Psychiatric Rating Scale.
*$P < .05$. **$P < .01$. ***$P < .001$. [a]$P < .1$.

Although both groups were reported at baseline to be markedly to severely ill, with no significant difference, there was a trend ($t = 1.85$, 26 df, $P < .08$) for the molindone group to be rated healthier at study end on the nurse-rated Clinical Global Impressions. The molindone group also was reported to have improved significantly more than the group on thioridazine ($t = 2.22$, $P < .035$). These are shown below in Table 5–6.

CPT results. All subjects quickly mastered the static or fixed mode CPT. Hit rates exceeded 96% for both drug groups, and false alarm rates remained below 3%. At the fixed ISI of 80 milliseconds, the P(A) ranged between 0.92 and 0.98. EOCs averaged 4%, far lower than those reported for inpatient children with disruptive disorders (Rapoport et al. 1980). There were no significant drug-placebo differences in these parameters, and no significant differences between the two medications.

The dynamic CPT showed a number of differences. In general, it overcame the "ceiling effect," producing lower hit rates, higher false alarm rates, and greater variability between subjects and sessions. The ISI increased significantly for molindone but not for thioridazine.

Table 5–6. Global Clinical Impressions nursing questionnaire (mean ± SD)

Item	Molindone (*N* = 15)	Thioridazine (*N* = 16)	*P*
How ill initially? (1 = well, 7 = highly ill)	5.33 ± 1.2	5.63 ± 1.3	NS
How ill at study end?	3.47 ± 0.6	4.13 ± 1.2	< .07
How much improved?	2.47 ± 0.7	3.18 ± 1.0	< .04
Therapeutic effect of drug?	3.4 ± 0.9	3.5 ± 0.7	NS
Side effects of drugs?	1.8 ± 0.94	1.67 ± 0.47	NS

The P(A) showed a mild, but not significant, elevation on thioridazine (compared with placebo), which agreed with improved attention in the classroom on the teacher's CTQ forms. There were no significant correlations between full-scale WISC-R scores and ISI or P(A). As shown in Table 5–7, the group on molindone showed the least CPT-related drug effects. The hit rate, false alarm rate, and P(A) did not vary for the molindone group, using either the standard CPT (static X) or the dynamic CPT. Carrying out dose-response curves across the group (not within individuals), molindone also did not show a medication effect on both types of the CPT. One criterion of a successful CPT run is the deterioration in performance over the course of a single CPT

Table 5–7. Dynamic Continuous Performance Test results

	Molindone (*N* = 15)		Thioridazine (*N* = 16)	
Side effect	**Placebo**	**On drug**	**Placebo**	**On drug**
Hit rate (%)	0.73	0.65	0.63	0.65
False alarm rate (%)	0.23	0.16	0.43	0.29
P(A)[a]	0.83	0.85	0.69	0.77*
Interstimulus interval (sec)	0.60	0.79*	0.84	0.66

[a]P(A) = estimated sensitivity based on signal detection theory.
*$P < .01$.

(Buchsbaum and Sostek 1980; Mackworth 1981). When CPT performance was repeated weekly, a mild practice effect was observed that led to mild but nonsignificant improvement, particularly for thioridazine for the dynamic CPT.

This effect mainly impacted on their false alarm rate, which may reflect the development of a more conservative style of responding, as suggested by Swets and Kristofferson (1970). This actually resulted in a nonsignificant improvement in the P(A), but without a separate placebo-treated control group it would be difficult to attribute it solely to medication treatment. Overall, there were no consistent correlations between drug dose, CPT variables (hit rate, EOCs, ISI), and any behavioral variables.

The dynamic CPT variables reported in this study show lower EOCs for our sample of inpatients with conduct disorder than for outpatient school-age children with ADHD (Rapoport et al. 1980). This may be due to the much higher proportion of targets in our dynamic CPT (25%) compared with those used in the Rapoport et al. study (5%). It may be that the rarity of actual targets leads to much more button presses in the Rapoport et al. sample. Even with this disparity, the ISI reported in our sample (58.2 milliseconds) is similar to that reported by Rapoport et al. in their treated ADHD sample.

Conclusions

The CPT procedures confirmed that the CPT with a fixed ISI showed ceiling effects, with all subjects performing well, regardless of drug status. The dynamic CPT, on the other hand, showed much lower hit rates and higher false alarm rates and met the criteria of Swets and Kristofferson (1970) that the task show a decline in performance over time. Even with the CPT procedure automatically adjusting itself to the patient's performance, only two difference were found. The group on thioridazine showed a trend for improved sensitivity, or P(A), when on drug, suggesting that their attentional performance did not deteriorate on medication. This is most interesting because the thioridazine group showed the highest rates of sedation on the DOTES. Conversely, the molindone group increased their mean ISI on medication, suggesting that their speed of performance had decreased while on medication. Both groups on drug were reported by the teacher to be more compliant and able to attend better, despite the findings on the CPT.

Our results are in general agreement with Klein (1991) regarding the minimal negative impact of neuroleptics on laboratory-measured cognitive functioning in children with psychiatric disorders. This is true even though she studied a different diagnostic group. We found no progressive disadvantage in laboratory-ascertained cognitive performance with continued inpatient neuroleptic treatment of children with severe conduct disorder.

One possibility for these discrepancies may be that the CPT is not very sensitive to neuroleptic drug effects. This is not surprising, for there have been no consistent findings about the impact of neuroleptics on a wide range of laboratory-based cognitive tests. Other than its effects on fine motor function found by both Klein (1991) and Platt et al. (1984), there may be no specific effects of neuroleptics. This would suggest that the CPT is most sensitive to stimulant-produced effects, whether negative or positive, and may be somewhat insensitive to neuroleptic effects.

Limitations of the Study

There were a number of limitations in this study. First, the fixed-flexible dosing scheme made it difficult to interpret the study findings because the ratings, taken at the last week on the fixed five-pill dosage, most likely showed carryover effects from the higher dosages taken during the flexible-dosing periods. This probably was truer for the thioridazine-treated children, given that the half-life of thioridazine is greater than it is for molindone. Second, there were significant IQ differences between the two groups, and this could mean that one group might be less apt at following instructions in completing the CPT. Indeed, some studies have shown significant correlations between CPT performance and IQ. We did not find such correlations. Third, the raters knew when the active neuroleptic was being given (although they were blind about which active drug was being given). As a result, the nurses and physician (but not the teacher) could be biased by expectancy effects and may have exaggerated differences between the active drug condition and the first or second placebo periods. Finally, we did not have a group of children who had been randomly assigned to placebo.

The use of the dynamic CPT in this study raises a number of concerns. As a measure, it has not continued to be employed in cognitive studies of pediatric psychopharmacology. The very nature of its self-correcting feedback loop raise concerns about its ability to study vigilance. What began as a solution to the problem of "ceiling effects" in the study of child patients proved to generate more problems than it solved. As Levy (1980) has shown, tasks of vigilance have a built-in developmental effect. Correcting the errors during the task itself makes it more difficult to link laboratory findings to the clinical classroom situation. The studies of Sykes et al. (1973) suggest when ADHD children are given shorter ISI intervals, and must perform faster, they actually have higher accuracy rates. This would suggest that any task that allowed the subject to select his or her own performance rate might not approximate the demands of a classroom or a vigilance task. It has been replaced by other approaches, which maintain the experimenter pacing of the original Rosvold et al. (1956) design but increase the difficulty of the task. Cornblatt et al. (1988) maintained a fixed ISI but revised the task demands to include matching pairs of complex signals, mixing signal types (each CPT run contains visual signals mixed with numerical targets, each consisting of four-number groupings) as well as using auditory distracters.

Clinical Implications

Evidence from laboratory measures can have considerable influence on practice, as well as publications and grant review committees. Laboratory measures utilizing a weight-adjusted dosing approach to aid data reduction have been carried uncritically into clinical practice. The dosing by weight standards of 0.3 mg/kg/dose for methylphenidate that followed a single publication (Sprague and Sleator 1977) that used a laboratory measure, the Paired Associates Task, became standard and customary in the treatment of ADHD children, even though it was not replicated by others and has been criticized (Rapport et al. 1990). In addition, group data often hide individual variations in treatment response that are likely to be encountered by the practitioner who works with one case at a time.

The prescribing of neuroleptics for children remains problematic for several reasons. Neuroleptics have broadband, nonspecific indications in childhood. Unlike other approved psychotropic medications, neuroleptics are listed in the 1991 *Physicians' Desk Reference* with symptomatic and behavioral, but not diagnostic, indications. Open, nonspecific indications leave much to the judgment of the clinician, even including the age limits, which extend down to the toddler phase of development.

Children on neuroleptics can develop short-term adverse treatment-emergent symptoms, such as acute dystonia, sedation (Gualtieri et al. 1980), weight gain (McAndrew et al. 1972; Planansky and Heilzer 1959), and even separation anxiety disorder and school refusal (Whitaker and Rao 1992). Longer-term problems, such as tardive dyskinesia, have also been reported (Gualtieri et al. 1980; Richardson et al. 1991). These side effects limit the usefulness of neuroleptics in the treatment of children with conduct disorders and rage outbursts (M. Campbell et al. 1992).

Although the sedating characteristics of these medications have long been known, the implications of potential cognitive impairment are a source of ongoing controversy. This study attempted to track cognitive changes related to neuroleptic medication usage in patients treated for 2 months with therapeutic doses of neuroleptics. One might infer that any medication with sedating effects would have the most impact on a test of sustained attention, such as the CPT. But, as indicated, the CPT may be rather insensitive to minor or moderate sedation, and the dynamic CPT may actually stimulate children with mild sedation, overcoming a problem that may occur in a classroom, where such constant reinforcement may not be available. Thus the use of any particular laboratory measure may not be relevant to other situations outside the research lab, such as the classroom, where medication-induced sedation or inability to concentrate may be more evident. Medication-related improvements and side effects for children must therefore be rated in several different domains to be clinically relevant.

References

Aman MG: Drugs, learning and psychotherapies, in Pediatric Psychopharmacology: The Use of Behavior Modifying Drugs With Children. Edited by Werry JS. New York, Brunner/Mazel, 1978, pp 79–108

American Psychiatric Association: Diagnostic and Statistical Manual of Mental Disorders, 3rd Edition. Washington, DC, American Psychiatric Association, 1980

Barker P, Fraser I: A controlled trial of haloperidol in children. Br J Psychiatry 114:855–857, 1968

Bergman A, Winters L, Cornblatt B: Methylphenidate: effects on sustained attention, in Ritalin: Theory and Patient Management. Edited by Greenhill LL, Osman B. New York, Mary Ann Liebert, 1991, pp 223–232

Buchsbaum MS, Sostek AJ: An adaptive-rate continuous performance test: vigilance characteristics and reliability for 400 male students. Percept Mot Skills 51:707–713, 1980

Campbell M, Fish B, Shapiro T, et al: Study of molindone in disturbed preschool children. Current Therapeutic Research 13:28–33, 1971

Campbell M, Cohen I, Small A: Drugs in aggressive behavior. Journal of the American Academy of Child Psychiatry 21:107–117, 1982a

Campbell M, Anderson L, Small A, et al: The effects of haloperidol and learning and behavior in autistic children. J Autism Dev Disord 12:167–175, 1982b

Campbell M, Small AM, Green WH, et al: Behavioral efficacy of haloperidol and lithium carbonate: a comparison in hospitalized aggressive children with conduct disorder. Arch Gen Psychiatry 41:650–656, 1984

Campbell M, Gonzales N, Silva R: The pharmacologic treatment of conduct disorders and rage outbursts. Psychiatr Clin North Am 15:69–87, 1992

Campbell SB, Douglas V, Morgenstern G: Cognitive styles in hyperactive children and the effect of methylphenidate. J Child Psychol Psychiatry 12:55–67, 1971

Claghorn JL: Review of clinical and laboratory experiences with molindone hydrochloride. J Clin Psychiatry 141:748–752, 1985

Conners K: Conners Rating Scale: use in clinical assessment, treatment planning, and research, in Use of Psychological Testing for Treatment Planning and Outcome Assessment. Edited by Marnish M. Hillside, NJ, Lawrence Erlbaum, 1994, pp 550–571

Cornblatt BA, Risch NJ, Faris G, et al: The Continuous Performance Test, Identical Pairs version (CPT-IP), I: new findings about sustained attention in normal families. Psychiatry Res 26:223–238, 1988

Crosby K: Attention and distractibility in mentally retarded and intellectually average children. American Journal of Mental Deficiency 77:46–53, 1972

Cunningham MA, Pillai V, Blachford-Rogers WJ: Haloperidol in the treatment of children with severe behavior disorders. Br J Psychiatry 114:845–854, 1968

Erlenmeyer-Kimling L, Cornblatt B: Attentional measures in a study of children at high-risk for schizophrenia. J Psychiatr Res 14:93–98, 1978

Gittelman-Klein R, Klein D, Katz S, et al: Comparative effects of methylphenidate and thioridazine in hyperkinetic children. Arch Gen Psychiatry 33:1217–1231, 1976

Goldstone S, Lhamon WT: The effects of haloperidol upon temporal information processing by patients with Tourette's syndrome. Psychopharmacology (Berlin) 50:7–10, 1976

Greenhill L, Barmack J, Spalten D, et al: Molindone hydrochloride in the treatment of aggressive, hospitalized children. Psychopharmacol Bull 17:125–127, 1981

Greenhill L, Solomon M, Pleak R, et al: Molindone hydrochloride treatment of hospitalized children with conduct disorder. J Clin Psychiatry 46:26–29, 1985

Gualtieri C, Barnhill J, McGimsey J, et al: Tardive dyskinesia and other movement disorders in children treated with psychotropic drugs. Journal of the American Academy of Child Psychiatry 19:491–510, 1980

Guy W: ECDEU Assessment Manual for Psychopharmacology, Revised (DHEW Publ No ADM-76-338). Rockville, MD, U.S. Department of Health, Education, & Welfare, 1976, pp 287–299, 383–394

Halperin JM, Wolf LE, Pascualvaca DM, et al: Differential assessment of attention and impulsivity in children. J Am Acad Child Adolesc Psychiatry 27:326–329, 1988

Halperin J, Sharma V, Greenblatt E, et al: Assessment of the continuous performance test: reliability and validity in a nonreferred sample. Psychological Assessment 3:603–608, 1991a

Halperin JM, Wolf L, Greenblatt ER, et al: Subtype analysis of commission errors on the continuous performance test in children. Developmental Neuropsychology 7:207–217, 1991b

Halperin JM, Newcorn JH, Sharma V: Ritalin: diagnostic comorbidity and attention measures, in Ritalin: Theory and Patient Management. Edited by Greenhill LL, Osman B. New York, Mary Ann Liebert, Inc, 1991, pp 15–14, 1991c

Halperin JM, Matier K, Bedi G, et al: Specificity of inattention, impulsivity, and hyperactivity to the diagnosis of attention-deficit hyperactivity disorder. J Am Acad Child Adolesc Psychiatry 31:190–196, 1992

Helper MM, Wilcott RC, Garfield SL: Effects of chlorpromazine on learning and related processes in emotionally disturbed children. J Consult Clin Psychol 27:1–9, 1963

Herman J, Mirsky AF, Ricks NL, et al: Behavioral and electrographic measures of attention in children at risk for schizophrenia. J Abnorm Psychol 86:27–33, 1977

Hollister L: Some human pharmacological studies of three psychotropic drugs: thiothixene, molindone, and W-1867. J Clin Pharmacol 8:190–195, 1968

Kagan J: Reflection-impulsivity: the generality of dynamics of conceptual tempo. J Abnorm Psychol 71:17–24, 1966

Kellner R, Rada R, Egelman A, et al: Long term study of molindone hydrochloride in chronic schizophrenia. Current Therapeutic Research 20:686–694, 1976

Klee SH, Garfinkel BD: The computerized continuous performance task: a new measure of inattention. J Abnorm Child Psychol 11:487–496, 1983

Klein RG: Thioridazine effects on the cognitive performance of children with attention-deficit hyperactivity disorder. Journal of Child and Adolescent Psychopharmacology 1:263–270, 1991

Klorman R, Bauer LO, Coons HW, et al: Enhancing effects of methylphenidate on normal young adults' cognitive processes. Psychopharmacol Bull 20:3–9, 1984

Kornetsky C, Mirsky AF, Kessler EK, et al: The effects of dextroamphetamine on behavioral deficits produced by sleep loss in humans. J Pharmacol Exp Ther 127:46–50, 1959

Kupietz S: Ritalin blood levels and their correlations with measures of learning, in Ritalin: Theory and Patient Management. Edited by Greenhill LL, Osman B. New York, Mary Ann Liebert, Inc, 1991, pp 247–255

Levy F: The development of sustained attention (vigilance) and inhibition in children: some normative data. J Child Psychol Psychiatry 21:77–84, 1980

Lipman R, DiMascio A, Reatig N, et al: Psychotropic drugs and mentally retarded children, in Psychopharmacology: A Generation of Progress. Edited by Lipton M, DiMascio A, Killam K. New York, Raven, 1978, pp 1437–1449

Mackworth JG: Performance decrement in vigilance, threshold, and high-speed perceptual motor tasks. Can J Psychol 17:302–325, 1981

McAndrew J, Case Q, Triffint D: Effects of prolonged phenothiazine intake on psychotic and other hospitalized subjects. Journal of Autism and Childhood Schizophrenia 2:75–91, 1972

Medical Economics: Physicians' Desk Reference, 45th Edition. Oradell, NJ, Medical Economics, 1991, pp 1951

Miller RG Jr: Simultaneous Statistical Inference, 2nd Edition. New York, Springer-Verlag, 1981

Nuechterlein KH: Signal detection in vigilance tasks and behavioral attributes among offspring of schizophrenic mothers and among hyperactive children. J Abnorm Psychol 92:4–28, 1983

Parasuraman R: Memory load and event rate control sensitivity decrements in sustained attention. Science 205:924–927, 1979

Planansky K, Heilzer F: Weight changes in relation to the characteristics of patients on chlorpromazine. Journal of Clinical and Experimental Psychopathology 20:53–57, 1959

Platt JE, Campbell M, Green WH, et al: Cognitive effects of lithium carbonate and haloperidol in treatment-resistant aggressive children. Arch Gen Psychiatry 41:657–662, 1984

Porteus SD: The Maze Test and Clinical Psychology. Palo Alto, CA, Pacific Books, 1959

Rapoport JL, Buchsbaum MS, Zahn TP, et al: Dextroamphetamine: cognitive and behavioral effects in normal prepubertal boys. Science 199:560–562, 1978

Rapoport JL, Buchsbaum MS, Weingartner H: Dextroamphetamine: cognitive and behavioral effects in normal and hyperactive children and normal adults. Arch Gen Psychiatry 37:933–943, 1980

Rapport M, DuPaul GJ, Kelly KL: Attention deficit hyperactivity disorder and methylphenidate: the relationship between gross body weight and drug response in children. Psychopharmacol Bull 25:285–290, 1989

Renshaw D: Mentally retarded, hyperkinetic, and psychotic children. Diseases of the Nervous System 38:575–576, 1977

Richardson M, Haugland G, Craig T: Neuroleptic use, parkinsonian symptoms, tardive dyskinesia and associated factors in child and adolescent psychiatric patients. Am J Psychiatry 148:1322–1328, 1991

Rosvold H, Mirsky A, Sarason I, et al: A continuous performance test of brain damage. Journal of Consulting Psychology 3:571–575, 1956

Rutschman J, Cornblatt B, Erlenmeyer-Kimling L: Sustained attention in children at risk for schizophrenia. Arch Gen Psychiatry 34:571–575, 1977

Sprague RL, Sleator EK: Methylphenidate in hyperkinetic children: differences in dose effects on learning and social behavior. Science 198:1274–1276, 1977

Sprague RL, Barnes KR, Werry JS: Methylphenidate and thioridazine: learning, reaction time, activity, and classroom behavior in disturbed children. Am J Orthopsychiatry 40:615–628, 1970

Swets JA, Kristofferson AB: Attention, in Annual Review of Psychology. Edited by Mussen PH, Rosenzweig MR. Palo Alto, CA, Annual Reviews, 1970

Sykes D, Douglas V, Weiss G, et al: Attention in hyperactive children and the effect of methylphenidate. J Child Psychol Psychiatry 12:129–139, 1971

Sykes D, Douglas V, Morgenstern G: The effect of methylphenidate on sustained attention in hyperactive children. Psychopharmacology (Berlin) 25:262–274, 1972

Sykes DH, Douglas VI, Morgenstern G: Sustained attention in hyperactive children. J Child Psychol Psychiatry 14:213–220, 1973

Teicher M, Glod C: Neuroleptic drugs: indications and guidelines for their rational use in children and adolescents. Journal of Child and Adolescent Psychopharmacology 1:33–56, 1990

Trites RL, Blouin AG, Laprade K: Factor analysis of the Conners Teacher Rating Scale based on a large normative sample. J Consult Clin Psychol 50:615–623, 1982

van der Meere J, Sergeant J: A divided attention experiment with pervasively hyperactive children. J Abnorm Child Psychol 15:379–392, 1987

Werry JS, Aman MG: Methylphenidate and haloperidol in children: effects on attention, memory, and activity. Arch Gen Psychiatry 32:790–795, 1975

Whalen C, Henker B, Collins BE, et al: A social ecology of hyperactive boys: medication effects in structured classroom environments. J Appl Behav Anal 12:65–81, 1979

Whitaker A, Rao U: Neuroleptics in pediatric psychiatry. Psychiatr Clin North Am 15:243–277, 1992

Winsberg BG, Yepes LE: Antipsychotics (major tranquilizers, neuroleptics), in Pediatric Psychopharmacology: The Use of Behavior Modifying Drugs With Children. Edited by Werry JS. New York, Brunner/Mazel, 1978, pp 214–273

Wong G, Cock R: Long-term effects of haloperidol on severally emotionally disturbed children. Aust N Z J Psychiatry 5:296–300, 1971

Zametkin AJ, Nordahl TE, Gross M, et al: Cerebral glucose metabolism in adults with hyperactivity of childhood onset. N Engl J Med 323:1361–1366, 1990

CHAPTER 6

Stereotypies and Neuroleptic-Related Dyskinesias in Children With Autism

Richard P. Malone, M.D.

In this chapter, the findings from studies in children with autism regarding two types of abnormal movement disorders are presented: stereotypies and neuroleptic-related dyskinesias. In describing the syndrome of autism, Kanner (1943) noted that children with this disorder displayed repetitive, rhythmic motor behaviors, including jumping in place, rocking, and twirling. A number of other motor behaviors, including teeth grinding, grimacing, hand flapping, finger movements, and toe walking, have been described (Freeman et al. 1981). These repetitive movements are known as stereotypies. Some of these stereotypies can be difficult to distinguish from neuroleptic-related dyskinesias (Meiselas et al. 1989; Shay et al. 1992). The similarities that exist between stereotypies and neuroleptic-related dyskinesias have implications for the use and monitoring of neuroleptics in the treatment of these children.

Stereotypies

Stereotypies are voluntary motor behaviors that are repetitive and purposeless and can involve any part of the body. Commonly encountered stereotypies in children with autism include rocking, twirling, hand flapping, and grimacing as well as a number of finer movements, especially in the orofacial area and in the distal extremities. These finer movements can include lip movements, mouth opening and closing, tongue protrusion and other tongue movements, eye closing and periorbital movements, finger twirling and finger twitches, and toe curling. Stereotypies can be seen in normal infants (Thelen 1979) as well as in a number of clinical conditions. Stereotypies have been described as a characteristic of some children who are blind (Troster et al. 1991) and some children who are deaf (Bachara and Phelan 1980). In persons with mental retardation, stereotypies can include destructive behaviors such as head banging and self-biting (American Psychiatric Association 1987).

Prevalence and Topography of Stereotypies in Children With Autism

Stereotypies occur almost universally in children with autism and can be seen in all body areas. Campbell et al. (1990) studied the relationship of stereotypies in children with autistic disorder. All 224 children were inpatients; their ages ranged from 2.32 to 8.22 years (mean, 4.61), with intellectual functioning ranging from low normal to severely retarded. They participated in a variety of pharmacological treatment studies and were rated at baseline before receiving any medication. Ratings were done twice at baseline employing a number of measures of abnormal movements, including the Abnormal Involuntary Movement Scale (AIMS) (National Institute of Mental Health 1985), the Abbreviated Dyskinesia Rating Scale (ADRS) (Simpson et al. 1979), and the Timed Stereotypies Rating Scale (TSRS) (Campbell 1985). The TSRS was specifically developed to rate the frequency and topography of stereotypies (Campbell and Palij 1985). In addition, the children were given behavioral ratings using the Children's Psychiatric Rating Scale (CPRS) (National Institute of Mental Health 1985), which contains an item for rating the presence and severity of stereotypies (item 28). Overall, 223 of the 224 subjects demonstrated at least mild stereotypies as rated by the CPRS at baseline. The severity of the stereotypies was negatively correlated with IQ on both the CPRS and the TSRS. Likewise, a number of other studies have demonstrated that IQ is inversely related to the presence of stereotypies in children with autism (Adrien et al. 1987; Bartak and Rutter 1976; Freeman et al. 1981). Baseline ratings (predrug) on the TSRS were available from 71 of the 224 subjects. On the TSRS, stereotypies were found in all body areas but most commonly in the orofacial area. Although stereotypies were identified more frequently in males than in females on the TSRS, no sex differences were found using the CPRS, and no relationship to age was demonstrated.

Effect of Neuroleptics on Stereotypies

Neuroleptics, which are dopamine antagonists, are among the most systematically studied drugs for the treatment of children with autism. Four separate double-blind and placebo-controlled studies of the short-term safety and efficacy of haloperidol in children with autism were completed (Anderson et al. 1984, 1989; Campbell et al. 1978; Cohen et al. 1980). In all, 135 children participated in these four studies. There were 102 males and 33 females ranging from ages 2.02 to 7.58 years. Haloperidol dosages ranged from 0.25 to 4.0 mg/day (12.5–200 chlorpromazine equivalents [CPZ-EQ]), or 0.016 to 0.217 mg/kg/day (see Table 6–1).

In three of the studies (Anderson et al. 1984, 1989; Campbell et al. 1978), the same measures were employed, including the CPRS. In the remaining study (Cohen et al. 1980), an interval recording measure containing an item for stereotypies was employed. Of those studies reporting on stereotypies specifically (Anderson et al. 1984; Campbell et al. 1978; Cohen et al. 1980), it was demonstrated that haloperidol, when compared with placebo, significantly decreased the severity of stereotypies. In the study of Anderson et al. (1989), the autism factor of the CPRS (see Overall and Campbell 1988), which includes stereotypies, was also significantly reduced. Some of the findings also suggested an age relationship in that haloperidol was more likely to decrease stereotypies in older than in younger children (Campbell et al. 1978; Cohen et al. 1980).

In addition to the effect on stereotypies, haloperidol was also shown to reduce a number of other symptoms, including withdrawal (Campbell et al. 1978; Cohen et al. 1980), hyperactivity, angry and labile affect, and abnormal relatedness (Anderson et

Table 6–1. Selected double-blind, placebo-controlled studies of haloperidol in children with autism

Reference	Total	*N*		Age (years)		Dosage (mg/day)		Dosage (mg/kg/day)	
		Males	Females	Range	Mean	Range	Mean	Range	Mean
Campbell et al. 1978	40	32	8	2.6–7.2	4.5	0.5–4.0	1.65	—	0.07[a]/ 0.15[b]
Cohen et al. 1980	10	6	4	2.1–7	4.7	1.0–4.0	1.65–1.9	—	—
Naruse et al. 1982[c]	34	—	—	3–16	—	0.75–6.75	—	—	—
Anderson et al. 1984	40	29	11	2.33–6.92	4.58	0.5–3.0	—	0.019–0.217	0.05
Anderson et al. 1989	45	35	10	2.02–7.59	4.49	0.25–4.0	0.844	0.016–0.184	0.047

[a]For subjects less than 4.5 years old.
[b]For subjects more than 4.5 years old.
[c]Haloperidol versus pimozide versus placebo.

al. 1984, 1989). Moreover, these studies demonstrated that learning was not impaired by the administration of haloperidol, but rather appeared to be facilitated (Anderson et al. 1984; Campbell et al. 1978; Cohen et al. 1980).

Naruse et al. (1982) compared the efficacy of haloperidol, pimozide, and placebo in 87 behaviorally disordered children, ages 3–16 years, 34 of whom were diagnosed with autism. In that study, haloperidol and pimozide were significantly better than placebo in reducing problem behaviors as measured by the Rating Scale for Abnormal Behavior in Children.

Several other classes of medications have been reported to affect the production of stereotypies in autistic children. Stimulant medications, which are dopamine agonists, have been reported to increase the production of stereotypies in some reports (Campbell et al. 1972b, 1976) but not all (Birmaher et al. 1988). The reports of Campbell et al. (1972b, 1976) indicated that not only could there be worsening of stereotypies, but also that stereotypies occurred de novo with administration of dextroamphetamine and levoamphetamine.

Fenfluramine, which decreases serotonin levels in autistic children (for review, see Aman and Kern 1989; Campbell 1988), has been demonstrated to decrease stereotypies in some studies (e.g., Campbell et al. 1988a; for review see Aman and Kern 1989) as has naltrexone, an opiate agonist (Campbell et al. 1988a, 1989a; Herman et al. 1986).

In this section, the issue of stereotypies that are a feature of autistic disorder was addressed. In the next section, neuroleptic-related dyskinesias are discussed. These involuntary abnormal movements are not a feature of autistic disorder, but rather an untoward effect of medication.

Neuroleptic-Related Dyskinesias in Children With Autism

As noted earlier, haloperidol has been demonstrated to be effective for the treatment of children with autistic disorder for a variety of behavioral problems, including decreasing stereotypies (see Campbell 1989 for review). In general, high-potency neuroleptics such as haloperidol are preferable to low-potency neuroleptics such as chlorpromazine or thioridazine because of the tendency of the lower-potency neuroleptics to cause sedation (Campbell et al. 1972a) and for chlorpromazine to decrease the seizure threshold (Tarjan et al. 1957). A major risk associated with neuroleptic use is the development of dyskinesias.

After demonstrating that haloperidol could be administered safely and effectively on a short-term basis in children with autism, it was necessary to investigate the safety and efficacy of haloperidol with longer-term administration. One of the critical issues for study for long-term haloperidol administration was the incidence of neuroleptic-related dyskinesias. Early studies reported that neuroleptic-related dyskinesias could be found in children who were exposed to neuroleptics. However, the reported prevalence of neuroleptic-related dyskinesias was quite broad, ranging from 8% to 51% (Campbell et al. 1983). A contributing factor to the broad range of reported prevalence was the number of methodological problems present in these studies, including a lack of baseline evaluation for abnormal movements, unspecified assessment measures, and treatment with multiple drugs.

The lack of a baseline assessment for abnormal movements was a critical flaw in these studies. As mentioned, most children with autism have a variety of stereotypies before exposure to any medications. These stereotypies often occur in the same body areas in which neuroleptic-related dyskinesias may later develop. The display of stereotypies can present difficulties in the evaluation of dyskinesias. As demonstrated in the studies mentioned earlier, neuroleptics decrease the severity of stereotypies. Therefore, when neuroleptics are discontinued, it is difficult to tell whether the movements that emerge represent the reappearance of baseline stereotypies or instead represent newly developed withdrawal dyskinesias. Moreover, at any point in time, not only at drug withdrawal, any abnormal movement that is demonstrated by an autistic child with a history of neuroleptic exposure could either be a stereotypy or a neuroleptic-related dyskinesia.

The early reports on neuroleptic-related dyskinesias often involved children with autism or mental retardation or both, and, presumably, many of these children would have had stereotypies at baseline before neuroleptics were administered. In these studies, neuroleptics were withdrawn and then the children were rated for the presence of neuroleptic-related dyskinesias (see Table 6–2). Clearly, an important methodological issue in withdrawal studies would be the ability of raters to distinguish between the reemergence of stereotypies and the emergence of withdrawal dyskinesias on discontinuation of neuroleptic. Addressing this issue, Meiselas et al. (1989) presented videotapes of 20 autistic children demonstrating either stereotypies or neuroleptic-related dyskinesias to three psychiatrists who were asked to rate blindly which of the two conditions was present. These 20 children were a subgroup of the children who participated in the long-term study of haloperidol in children with autism. Two of the raters were research psychiatrists, experts in rating tardive dyskinesia, and the third was a clinician with experience in evaluating and treating children with autism. These experienced psychiatrists had difficulty distinguishing stereotypies from neuroleptic-related dyskinesias. This finding suggests that the early studies of neuroleptic-related dyskinesias in children may not have accurately reported the prevalence of dyskinesias because the raters may not have been able to differentiate the two

Table 6–2. Selected studies of dyskinesias in children with developmental disabilities

Reference	*N*	Age range (years)	Design	Incidence of dyskinesias (%)
McAndrew et al. 1972	125	4–16	Withdrawal, retrospective	8
Polizos and Engelhardt 1978	53	8.8[a]	Withdrawal, retrospective	51
Gualtieri et al. 1984	41	3–21	Withdrawal, retrospective	44
Gualtieri et al. 1986	38	5–57	Withdrawal, retrospective	34
Campbell et al. 1989b	104	2–8	Prospective	27

[a]Mean.

abnormal movements (i.e., stereotypies and neuroleptic-related dyskinesias).

A Prospective Study of Haloperidol in Children With Autism

Design

A study on long-term haloperidol administration overcame many of the above-mentioned methodological problems. Importantly, the study was prospective, and subjects were rated at baseline before exposure to the neuroleptic. All of the 104 subjects met DSM-III (American Psychiatric Association 1980) criteria for infantile autism. The subjects were a subset of those from the study on stereotypies mentioned earlier (Campbell et al. 1988b, 1990) consisting of 82 males and 22 females ranging in age from 2.32 to 8.22 years. Their intellectual functioning ranged from low average to severely retarded. All were inpatients at the Therapeutic Nursery at Bellevue Hospital, New York, for the initial regulation of haloperidol and then followed as outpatients. To ensure that any abnormal movements seen at baseline were stereotypies, subjects were excluded from the study when they had either a history of chronic neuroleptic exposure (although most had *no* prior exposure to psychotropic medications) or any history of neuroleptic-related dyskinesias. Thus, a baseline record of stereotypies was available for each subject, and this record could be employed later in distinguishing stereotypies from neuroleptic-related dyskinesias. Importantly, each of the rating sessions was videotaped, providing a permanent recording that could be reviewed at a later time.

Haloperidol dosage was individually regulated to obtain optimal therapeutic benefit while minimizing untoward effects. Medication was begun following 2 weeks of baseline measures and was then continued for the next 6 months. After 6 months of treatment, the medication was discontinued, and all subjects were placed on open placebo for 4 weeks. Every effort was made to keep the dosage of medication for a given patient constant during the 6-month treatment period. At the end of the placebo period, subjects who continued to require haloperidol treatment were restarted on medication and reentered the active phase of the study.

As in the short-term studies, the following measures were employed: the AIMS, the ADRS, and the CPRS. Rating sessions were videotaped during the baseline assessment period and during the 4 weeks of posttreatment placebo administration. Additionally, the children returned at least monthly for a medication review. At that time, they were rated for abnormal movements employing the AIMS procedure, and caretakers were questioned regarding any abnormal movements observed in the intervening times.

Details and discussion of these structured videotaped rating sessions can be found elsewhere (Campbell and Palij 1985; Campbell et al. 1978, 1988b). Briefly, each child was seen at a fixed time in the morning for a 20-minute evaluative session, following medication. During this session, each child performed various tasks from the Gesell (Gesell and Amatruda 1946), a measure of developmental level, followed by the AIMS procedure. Ratings were made based on behaviors displayed during the session. The baseline videotape recordings were later employed in the evaluation of abnormal movements, particularly when it was not clear if the movement being displayed was present at baseline. To reiterate, baseline movements that decreased on haloperidol could reemerge after withdrawal of the drug, which is the same time when withdrawal dyskinesias emerge. When a question arose concerning an abnormal movement, the baseline record and videotape were reviewed. If the exact abnormal movement was seen at baseline, the movement would not be rated as a neuroleptic-related dyskinesia and would be considered a baseline movement not related to medication. However, if the movement was not present at baseline or had a markedly different frequency or severity, it would likely be rated as a neuroleptic-related dyskinesia. Neuroleptic-related dyskinesias were diagnosed clinically and employing the research criteria of Schooler and Kane (1982).

Findings From the Long-Term Study

Haloperidol continued to be effective when administered on a long-term basis, particularly for children with prominent behavioral symptoms such as irritability, anger, labile affect, and uncooperativeness (Perry et al. 1989). Optimal haloperidol dosages ranged from 0.5 to 4.0 mg/day (25–200 CPZ-EQ), and no sedation or parkinsonian side effects were observed at optimal dosage. The medication was equally effective whether the dosage was administered on a continuous schedule (daily) or a discontinuous schedule (5 of 7 days/week) for a period of 6 months (Perry et al. 1989).

Overall, 29 (27.9%) of 104 subjects who participated in the study for a period of at least 6 months of drug followed by placebo and up to 10 such periods developed neuroleptic-related dyskinesias at least once (Malone et al. 1991). In 24 (82.8%) of these 29 subjects, neuroleptic-related dyskinesias were first observed when haloperidol was discontinued; in the remaining 5 subjects, the neuroleptic-related dyskinesias were first observed during haloperidol administration. All of the neuroleptic-related dyskinesias were found to be reversible within 16 days to 7.5 months.

In adult populations, a number of possible risk factors for developing neuroleptic-related dyskinesias have been identified, although only older age and female sex have been consistently demonstrated across studies (for a review, see Kane and Smith 1982). However, attempts at establishing risk factors in children who develop neuroleptic-related dyskinesias have been largely unsuccessful. To date, none of the following variables differentiate those children who develop neuroleptic-related dyskinesias: age, weight, IQ, clinical symptoms, cumulative dosage, or length of haloperidol exposure (Campbell et al. 1988b). At an early point in the study, female sex seemed to be a possible risk factor for developing neuroleptic-related dyskinesia in children with autism (Campbell et al. 1988b), but this finding "washed out" as the study continued (Campbell et al. 1989b).

The topography of neuroleptic-related dyskinesias was similar to that described earlier for stereotypies in that they were found in all body areas but most commonly in the orofacial area (Campbell et al. 1988b, 1990). Although stereotypies and neuroleptic-related dyskinesias have a similar distribution, baseline measures of stereotypies have not been related to the later development of neuroleptic-related dyskinesias (Locascio et al. 1991).

Repeated Dyskinesias

A number of children who developed neuroleptic-related dyskinesias continued to require haloperidol for clinical reasons and were placed back on medication, remaining in the study for up to 10 cycles of 6 months of haloperidol and placebo administration. Of the 29 subjects who developed neuroleptic-related dyskinesias, 15 did not develop dyskinesias again in the course of the study (Malone et al. 1991). Of these 15 children, 10 were dropped from the study for a variety of reasons and not placed back on haloperidol. Therefore, for those 10 children, further follow-up on haloperidol was not available. The remaining 5 did receive further haloperidol treatment without developing dyskinesias again.

Of the 29 children who developed dyskinesias, 14 demonstrated reversible neuroleptic-related dyskinesias that recurred *multiple times* during the study (Malone et al. 1991). Because the study included both an active haloperidol treatment phase and a later withdrawal phase, neuroleptic-related dyskinesias could be observed both on drug and on withdrawal of drug. Seven subjects had withdrawal dyskinesias in at least three different placebo periods during the study. To investigate changes that may occur when withdrawal dyskinesias are demonstrated repeatedly, these data were further analyzed. Repeated-measures analysis of variance showed that when withdrawal dyskinesias recurred, they tended to appear sooner after drug withdrawal (13.0 ± 7.5 days versus 12.0 ± 7.8 days versus 5.0 ± 3.4 days, $F = 11.29$, $P < .05$) and to last for a longer time (17.4 ± 13.8 days versus 71.1 ± 60.6 days versus 53.1 ± 36.5 days, $F = 5.94$, $P < .05$) (Malone et al. 1991).

Overall, dyskinesias were seen more often on discontinuation of medication than they were while the child was on the drug. Of the 14 children, 8 demonstrated neuroleptic-related dyskinesias only in the withdrawal phase; the remaining 6 children demonstrated neuroleptic-related dyskinesias during both the withdrawal phase and with active treatment (4 of these 6 had withdrawal dyskinesias first). No variables, including age, sex, or IQ, distinguished those subjects who never developed dyskinesias from those who developed dyskinesias once or multiple times.

Because of the small sample size it is difficult to generalize these results to other populations. Yet, these data are valuable in that there is no other prospective study of neuroleptic-related dyskinesias in children with autism. There is a suggestion that withdrawal dyskinesias increase in severity with regard to earlier time at onset and longer duration when children remain on medication. However, not all children who develop withdrawal dyskinesias once will develop them again. The relationship between developing withdrawal dyskinesias and developing dyskinesias on drug remains unclear, but it does seem that the withdrawal-emergent dyskinesias are usually observed before the treatment-emergent dyskinesias.

Conclusions

Stereotypies and neuroleptic-related dyskinesias are abnormal movement disorders that can be seen in children with autism. Some of these movements are similar in their manifestations. Stereotypies are a characteristic feature of the disorder, occurring in most children with autism. Neuroleptic-related dyskinesias are an untoward effect of medication and occur in approximately 29% of autistic children treated with neuroleptics.

It has been demonstrated that neuroleptics reduce stereotypies. On discontinuation of neuroleptic treatment, stereotypies that had been suppressed with medication may reemerge. Likewise, neuroleptic-related dyskinesias are seen more frequently on discontinuation of medication than they are during active treatment (Campbell et al. 1988b; Malone et al. 1991). In that both stereotypies and neuroleptic-related dyskinesias are similar in appearance and topography, it can be particularly difficult to distinguish stereotypies from dyskinesias, especially if an abnormal movement occurs when medication is discontinued. Therefore, it is critical to document the presence of stereotypies or any other abnormal movements at baseline, before neuroleptic treatment is instituted in children with autism. Should abnormal movements be noted after the institution of neuroleptics, this baseline record of stereotypies could be employed to help differentiate stereotypies from dyskinesias.

The studies reported in this chapter suggest that in some children withdrawal dyskinesias occur sooner and have a longer duration when neuroleptics continue to be administered. The clinician's task remains difficult, however, because risk factors for developing neuroleptic-related dyskinesias in children with autism have not yet been clearly identified. However, with improved rating techniques, including the use of videotapes and standard rating scales, future studies of this population may provide the necessary keys to this troubling aspect of neuroleptic treatment.

References

Adrien JL, Ornitz E, Barthelemy C, et al: The presence or absence of certain behaviors associated with infantile autism in severely retarded autistic and nonautistic retarded children and very young normal children. J Autism Dev Disord 17:407–416, 1987

Aman MG, Kern RA: Review of fenfluramine in the treatment of the developmental disabilities. J Am Acad Child Adolesc Psychiatry 28:549–565, 1989

American Psychiatric Association: Diagnostic and Statistical Manual of Mental Disorders, 3rd Edition. Washington, DC, American Psychiatric Association, 1980

American Psychiatric Association: Diagnostic and Statistical Manual of Mental Disorders, 3rd Edition, Revised. Washington, DC, American Psychiatric Association, 1987

Anderson LT, Campbell M, Grega DM, et al: Haloperidol in the treatment of infantile autism: effects on learning and behavioral symptoms. Am J Psychiatry 141:1195–1202, 1984

Anderson LT, Campbell M, Adams P, et al: The effects of haloperidol on discrimination learning and behavioral symptoms in autistic children. J Autism Dev Disord 19:227–239, 1989

Bachara GH, Phelan WJ: Rhythmic movement in deaf children. Percept Mot Skills 50:933–934, 1980

Bartak L, Rutter M: Differences between mentally retarded and normally intelligent autistic children. Journal of Autism and Childhood Schizophrenia 6:109–120, 1976

Birmaher B, Quintana H, Greenhill LL: Case study: methylphenidate treatment of hyperactive autistic children. J Am Acad Child Adolesc Psychiatry 27:248–251, 1988

Campbell M: Timed stereotypies rating scale. Psychopharmacol Bull 21:1082, 1985

Campbell M: Fenfluramine treatment of autism. J Child Psychol Psychiatry 29:1–10, 1988

Campbell M: Pharmacotherapy in autism: an overview, in Diagnosis and Treatment of Autism. Edited by Gillberg C. New York, Plenum, 1989, pp 203–217

Campbell M, Palij M: Behavioral and cognitive measures used in psychopharmacological studies of infantile autism. Psychopharmacol Bull 21:1047–1053, 1985

Campbell M, Fish B, Korein J, et al: Lithium and chlorpromazine: a controlled crossover study of hyperactive severely disturbed young children. Journal of Autism and Childhood Schizophrenia 2:234–263, 1972a

Campbell M, Fish B, David R, et al: Response to triiodothyronine and dextroamphetamine: a study of preschool schizophrenic children. Journal of Autism and Childhood Schizophrenia 2:343–358, 1972b

Campbell M, Small AM, Collins PJ, et al: Levodopa and levoamphetamine: a crossover study in young schizophrenic children. Current Therapeutic Research 19:70–86, 1976

Campbell M, Anderson LT, Meier M, et al: A comparison of haloperidol, behavior therapy and their interaction in autistic children. J Am Acad Child Adolesc Psychiatry 17:640–655, 1978

Campbell M, Grega DM, Green WH, et al: Neuroleptic-induced dyskinesias in children. Clin Neuropharmacol 6:207–222, 1983

Campbell M, Adams P, Small AM, et al: Efficacy and safety of fenfluramine in autistic children. J Am Acad Child Adolesc Psychiatry 27:434–439, 1988a

Campbell M, Adams P, Perry R, et al: Tardive and withdrawal dyskinesia in autistic children: a prospective study. Psychopharmacol Bull 24:251–255, 1988b

Campbell M, Overall JE, Small AM, et al: Naltrexone in autistic children: an acute open dose range tolerance trial. J Am Acad Child Adolesc Psychiatry 28:200–206, 1989a

Campbell M, Malone RP, Perry R, et al: Neuroleptic-related dyskinesias in autistic children, in Scientific Proceedings, Vol V, 36th Annual Meeting, American Academy of Child and Adolescent Psychiatry, New York, New York, October 11–15, 1989b, p 67

Campbell M, Locascio JJ, Choroco MC, et al: Stereotypies and tardive dyskinesia: abnormal movements in autistic children. Psychopharmacol Bull 26:260–266, 1990

Cohen IL, Campbell M, Posner D, et al: Behavioral effects of haloperidol in young autistic children: an objective analysis using a within-subjects reversal design. Journal of the American Academy of Child Psychiatry 19:665–677, 1980

Freeman BJ, Ritvo ER, Schroth PC, et al: Behavioral characteristics of high- and low-IQ autistic children. Am J Psychiatry 138:25–29, 1981

Gesell A, Amatruda C: Developmental Diagnosis. Hagerstown, MD, Harper & Row, 1946

Gualtieri CT, Quade D, Hicks RE, et al: Tardive dyskinesia and other clinical consequences of neuroleptic treatment in children and adolescents. Am J Psychiatry 141:20–23, 1984

Gualtieri CT, Schroeder SR, Hicks RE, et al: Tardive dyskinesia in young mentally retarded individuals. Arch Gen Psychiatry 43:335–340, 1986

Herman BH, Hammock MK, Arthur-Smith A, et al: Effects of naltrexone in autism: correlation with plasma opioid concentrations. Scientific Proceedings for the Annual Meeting of the AACAP 2:11–12, 1986

Kane JM, Smith JM: Tardive dyskinesia: prevalence and risk factors, 1959 to 1979. Arch Gen Psychiatry 39:473–481, 1982

Kanner L: Autistic disturbances of affective contact. Nervous Child 2:217–250, 1943

Locascio JJ, Malone RP, Small AM, et al: Factors related to haloperidol response and dyskinesias in autistic children. Psychopharmacol Bull 27:119–126, 1991

Malone RP, Ernst M, Godfrey KA, et al: Repeated episodes of neuroleptic-related dyskinesias in autistic children. Psychopharmacol Bull 27:113–117, 1991

McAndrew JB, Case Q, Treffert DA: Effects of prolonged phenothiazine intake on psychotic and other hospitalized children. Journal of Autism and Childhood Schizophrenia 2:75–91, 1972

Meiselas KD, Spencer EK, Oberfield R, et al: Differentiation of stereotypies from neuroleptic-related dyskinesias in autistic children. J Clin Psychopharmacol 9:207–209, 1989

Naruse H, Nagahata M, Nakane Y, et al: A multicenter double-blind trial of pimozide (Orap), haloperidol and placebo in children with behavior disorders, using crossover design. Acta Paedopsychiatrica 48:173–184, 1982

National Institute of Mental Health: Rating scales and assessment instruments for use in pediatric psychopharmacology research (special feature). Psychopharmacol Bull 21:765–770, 1985

Overall JE, Campbell M: Behavioral assessment of psychopathology in children: infantile autism. J Clin Psychol 44:708–716, 1988

Perry R, Campbell M, Adams P, et al: Long-term efficacy of haloperidol in autistic children: continuous versus discontinuous drug administration. J Am Acad Child Adolesc Psychiatry 28:87–92, 1989

Polizos P, Engelhardt DM: Dyskinetic phenomena in children treated with psychotropic medications. Psychopharmacol Bull 14:65–68, 1978

Schooler NR, Kane JM: Research diagnoses for tardive dyskinesia. Arch Gen Psychiatry 39:486–487, 1982

Shay J, Sanchez LE, Cueva JE, et al: Neuroleptic-related dyskinesias and stereotypies in autistic children: videotape ratings. Abstracts of 31st Annual Meeting, American College of Neuropharmacology, San Juan, Puerto Rico, December 14–18, 1992

Simpson GM, Lee JH, Zoubok B, et al: A rating scale for tardive dyskinesia. Psychopharmacology (Berlin) 64:171–179, 1979

Tarjan C, Lowry VE, Wright SW: Use of chlorpromazine in two hundred seventy-eight mentally deficient patients. AMA Journal of Disturbed Children 94:294–300, 1957

Thelen E: Rhythmical stereotypies in normal human infants. Animal Behavior 27:699–715, 1979

Troster H, Brambring M, Beelmann A: Prevalence and situational causes of stereotyped behaviors in blind infants and preschoolers. J Abnorm Child Psychol 19:569–590, 1991

CHAPTER 7

Treatment of Tic Disorders With Neuroleptic Drugs

Arthur K. Shapiro, M.D.
Elaine Shapiro, Ph.D.

In this chapter, we evaluate the effectiveness of neuroleptic drugs and provide guidelines for the treatment of children with tic disorders and Tourette's disorder or syndrome (TS). It relies primarily on controlled studies and, when such data are unavailable, on other clinical research, the authors' experience in the evaluation and treatment of more than 3,600 patients since 1965, and a comprehensive study of 666 patients (A. K. Shapiro et al. 1988).

History of Tic Disorders

The first retrospective description of a person with possible TS is a priest described in the *Malleus Maleficarum* by Kramer and Sprenger in 1489 (1971). Other possible examples cited are an adult female in 1663 and a family of barking girls in 1701 (Lees 1985), Prince de Conde in the 17th century (Stevens 1971), and Samuel Johnson in the 18th century (Boswell 1791; McHenry 1967; Murray 1979, 1982). The first full description of a patient with TS was by Itard (1825) of the Marquise du Dampiere. She was later one of the nine patients described by Gilles de la Tourette (1885). Trousseau (1873) briefly but relevantly described some of the symptoms of TS, then referred to as "maladie des tics." But it was not until Gilles de la Tourette published his classic article that "Tourette's syndrome" (now called "Tourette's disorder" in the United States) became an established disorder.

Despite Tourette's astute description of the symptoms, the disorder was massively underdiagnosed up to the middle of the 1970s, related to errors in the diagnostic criteria and to the belief that the etiology was psychological and required psychological treatment. For example, only 50 cases were identified in a review of the English-language literature by 1965 (Fernando 1967). With development of a data orientation in medicine and psychiatry, reliable and valid criteria for the diagnosis of tic disorders, evidence for a biological etiology, and effective treatment with neuroleptics, the number of identified cases increased dramatically. It is now apparent that tic disorders are much more frequent than previously imagined. An epidemiological survey in Japan estimated a prevalence of 5.1% for transient tic disorder, 2.2% for chronic motor tic disorder, and 0.5% for TS (Nomoto and Machiyama 1990).

Characteristics of Tic Disorders

Tics are defined as involuntary movements, vocalizations, or sensations that have been described variously as rapid, brief, quick, sudden, ejaculatory, recurrent, repetitive, stereotypic, nonrhythmic, occurring at irregular intervals, purposeless, inappropriate, irresistible, and either simple or complex. Transient tic disorder is diagnosed if the symptoms disappear within a year of onset. If the symptoms last more than a year, the diagnosis is chronic motor tic disorder if only muscular symptoms are present, or chronic vocal tic disorder if only vocal tics are present. For a diagnosis of TS, both muscular and vocal symptoms must be present sometime during the course of the illness for more than a year. Tic disorder not otherwise specified is reserved for a tic disorder that does not meet the criteria for a specific tic disorder. Some patients have a sensory tic subtype that consists of dysphoric sensations that result in voluntary squeezes or dystonic movements (Kurlan et al. 1989; A. K. Shapiro and Shapiro 1992; A. K. Shapiro et al. 1988). The symptoms wax, wane, and fluctuate over time, and diverse stimuli can increase or decrease the occurrence of tics. It should be emphasized that not every movement, noise, or obscenity is a tic, and tics have to be differentiated from habits, mannerisms, compulsions, stereotypic symptoms, and diverse organic symptoms. Moreover, there are other movement disorders of undetermined etiology that currently defy classification and frequently do not respond to treatment with neuroleptics (A. K. Shapiro et al. 1988).

The average age at onset for a tic disorder is 6–7 years; 90% of patients have an onset by age 10, 99% by age 14, and usually before age 21. More than 90% of patients—and more than 60% of patients in specialty clinics—are estimated to have very mild symptoms. All patients report spontaneous waxing, waning, and fluctuation of symptoms over time. Diagnostic criteria, essentially similar to the criteria in DSM-III-R (American Psychiatric Association 1987), have been developed by a consensus committee and incorporated in DSM-IV (American Psychiatric Association 1994).

Although controversial, our conclusion is that tic disorders and TS are not associated with other behavioral, psychological, or medical disorders and that the appropriate treatment for a tic disorder that induces psychosocial distress is the use of medication to minimize tic symptoms. Other problems should be evaluated separately and treated using appropriate medications. For example, neuroleptics are effective for the treatment of tics or TS, stimulants for attention-deficit/hyperactivity disorder (ADHD), and antiobsessional drugs for obsessive-compulsive symptoms or disorder (OCS-OCD) (A. K. Shapiro and Shapiro 1992; A. K. Shapiro et al. 1988).

Effectiveness of Medication

Historically, it seems that every known drug and procedure has been used to treat TS: religious treatment such as exorcism and Christian Science; procedures such as cathartics, enemas, emetics, bleeding and other methods of dehydration, hydrotherapy, cold, hot, and tepid douches, warm fomentations, electricity, rhythmic traction of the tongue, thoracic compression, phrenic electricization, static sparks, diet, nutrition, massage, isolation, seclusion, rest, and exercise; drugs such as homeopathic remedies, conium, bromides, chloral hydrate, opium, morphine, laudanum, the basic extract, curare, chloroform, ether, zinc valerianate, valerian, gelsemium, quinine, cannabis indican, arsenic, mustard plasters, cocaine, kola, coca, condurango, blanco, cimicufuga nigra, opioids, sedatives, hypnotics, and minor and major tranquilizers; electric and insulin convulsive treatment; surgical treatment such as tonsillectomy, elongation, section, cautery to the vertebral column, or ligature of the spinal accessory nerve, resection of the trigeminal and spinofacial anastomoses, lobotomies, cryothalamectomy, and chemothalamectomy; and all manner of psychological treatment from psychoanalysis to Erhard Seminars Training (EST) (A. K. Shapiro et al. 1988).

This disparate history began to change after 1961 following the successful use of haloperidol in single patients with TS by Seignot (1961) in France and by Caprini and Melotti (1961) in Italy. A discussion of several classes of drugs and specific medications currently used to treat TS follows.

Butyrophenones

Haloperidol

Haloperidol has been extensively used to treat patients with TS (A. K. Shapiro et al. 1978; E. Shapiro et al. 1989). Based on clinical reports and the results of several uncontrolled studies, the Food and Drug Administration (FDA) approved haloperidol for the treatment of adult patients with TS in 1969 and for children in 1978. Despite the long use of haloperidol, the first adequately controlled study supporting the effectiveness of haloperidol was not published until 1989 (E. Shapiro et al. 1989).

Haloperidol has been reported to improve 62%–91% of patients and has become the drug of choice for the treatment of TS (Borison et al. 1982; Golden 1977b; Nee et al. 1980; Nomura and Segawa 1979; A. K. Shapiro et al. 1973, 1978, 1988; E. Shapiro et al. 1989; Wassman et al. 1978). Some clinicians, however, report less favorable results (D. J. Cohen et al. 1980; Ford and Gottlieb 1969; Leckman et al. 1982; Tibbits 1981; Van Woert et al. 1982). Anecdotal reports that haloperidol is more effective than phenothiazines is possibly related to its ability to bind more specifically to D_2 than to D_1 receptors. Haloperidol also has some adrenergic (alpha-1) antagonistic activity that may account for some of its akinesic or sedative adverse effects.

Our clinical impressions indicate that 25% of patients have at least 80% reduction of symptoms at a low dosage without significant adverse effects. Another 50% of patients develop adverse effects when treated with therapeutic dosages of haloperidol, but these can be managed successfully over time. The remaining 25% are treatment failures, usually because adverse effects nullify therapeutic benefit, or, in retrospect, it is found that the patient had another nontic type of movement disorder. The general consensus among clinicians is that haloperidol is an effective treatment for the symptoms of TS.

Diphenylbutylpiperidines

Pimozide

Pimozide is reported selectively to block central dopamine receptors, preferentially to bind to dopamine D_2 receptors (Casamenti et al. 1980; Goldberg 1985), and to have little effect on norepinephrine receptors (Anden et al. 1970; Matthysse 1973; Nose and Takemoto 1975; Nyback et al. 1970; Peroutka et al. 1977; Seeman and Lee 1975). Controlled studies confirmed the effectiveness of pimozide for the treatment of TS (Ross and Moldofsky 1978; A. K. Shapiro and Shapiro 1984) and led to its approval by the FDA for the treatment of TS under the Orphan Drug Act in 1984.

The clinical literature provides some evidence that pimozide may be more effective and may have a lower potential for akinesic or sedative adverse effects than haloperidol (Debray et al. 1972; Nomura and Segawa 1982; Opler and Feinberg 1991; Ross and Moldofsky 1978; A. K. Shapiro and Shapiro 1984; A. K. Shapiro et al. 1983a, 1987). However, these were not confirmed in the previously cited controlled study of haloperidol and pimozide (E. Shapiro et al. 1989). Both drugs were significantly better than placebo, but there was essentially no difference between the two drugs, and adverse effects were slightly more frequent for pimozide. Limitations of the study include the use of a restricted dosage for pimozide mandated by the FDA and the short duration of treatment of 6 weeks for each drug category. Regeur et al. (1986) followed up 33 patients who had been treated with 2–18 mg of pimozide (67–600 mg chlorpromazine equivalents [CPZ-EQ]) and 2–15 mg of haloperidol (100–750 mg CPZ-EQ) for 1–5 years and reported both to be effective, but significantly fewer patients treated with pimozide discontinued treatment compared with patients treated with haloperidol.

Overall, both clinical and experimental evidence indicates that haloperidol and pimozide have a similar effectiveness and adverse effects profile, with some specificity by patient.

Penfluridol

Although not available in the United States, penfluridol, a long-lasting diphenylbutylpiperidine, is thought to be a specific blocker of dopamine without significant norepinephrine or 5-hydroxytryptamine blocking effects (Nose and Takemoto 1975; Seeman and Lee 1975). This mode of action may result in more improvement than with haloperidol and fewer and less severe akinesic, sedative, depressive, dysphoric, motivational, and cognitive adverse effects.

These speculations are supported by open clinical trials of a small number of patients: 7 patients (Holomboe 1977), 1 patient (Parikh et al. 1979), and 15 patients (A. K. Shapiro et al. 1983b, 1988). The results of these open, uncontrolled clinical studies suggest that penfluridol may be a worthwhile alternative drug for the treatment of TS, yielding more improvement and less akinesic adverse effects than haloperidol. An additional advantage of penfluridol is weekly or biweekly administration. However, pancreatic and mammary tumors have been reported in studies of rats given high oral dosages of penfluridol. Although the significance of these findings for humans is unknown and there are no reliable published reports of carcinogenesis for any neuroleptic, the FDA and McNeil Pharmaceuticals discontinued investigatory use of penfluridol in the United States, although it is available in many other countries.

Phenothiazines

Fluphenazine

Fluphenazine was reported as effective but with fewer adverse effects than haloperidol in an open study of 21 patients (Goetz et al. 1984). In a briefly described, double-blind, controlled study of 10 patients, patients were treated with fluphenazine, trifluoperazine, and haloperidol. All three agents were judged to be equally effective, but fluphenazine had fewer adverse effects (Borison et al. 1982). This study was limited, however, in that the sample size was too small to have the statistical power necessary to demonstrate differences among the neuroleptics in a crossover design. Other limitations of this study were the failure to report previous treatment, whether the patients were haloperidol resisters, the length of the therapeutic trial, and whether medication was used to control adverse effects. In a retrospective review of 31 patients treated with fluphenazine and 60 with haloperidol, good to fair improvement was reported by 81% of patients on fluphenazine and by 83% of patients on haloperidol, but fluphenazine had fewer adverse effects (Singer et al. 1986).

Although these studies suggest that fluphenazine and possibly trifluoperazine induce fewer adverse effects than haloperidol, confirmatory controlled studies that utilize adequate sample sizes and exclusion of resisters to haloperidol treatment are warranted. Our clinical impression is that haloperidol, pimozide, and fluphenazine are equally effective and induce similar adverse effects in most patients. However, some patients obtain more benefit or less adverse effects by a change from one of these drugs to the other.

Other Phenothiazines

Favorable clinical response is occasionally reported for treatment with phenothiazines such as chlorpromazine and thiopropazate (A. K. Shapiro et al. 1988). Our clinical experience suggests that these phenothiazines are less effective overall compared with haloperidol and pimozide. However, carefully controlled clinical trials are needed to clarify this clinical impression. The major limitations of the phenothiazines are akinesia, photosensitivity, seizures, dermatitis, and blood and liver dyscrasias for the aliphatic group such as chlorpromazine; significantly more extrapyramidal symptoms such as akathisia, akinesia, dyskinesia, and parkinsonism for the piperazine subgroup such as trifluoperazine, perphenazine, and prochlorperazine; and increased sedative and sexual adverse effects in the piperidyl group such as thioridazine.

The pattern of adverse effects for the butyrophenones and diphenylbutylpiperidines are similar to the piperazine subgroup of phenothiazines.

Miscellaneous Dopamine Antagonists

Tetrabenazine

Tetrabenazine is a benzoquinolizine derivative that depletes brain storage of catecholamines. Fourteen patients were treated by us in an open study with oral dosages up to 300 mg/day (A. K. Shapiro et al. 1978). Initial improvement in 12 patients, associated with sedation and akinesia, was not sustained after 2 months (A. K. Shapiro et al. 1978, 1988; Sweet et al. 1974). However, a more positive result is reported in an open trial of nine patients who were treated an average of 9.4 months (1–20 months) with dosages that ranged from 25 to 100 mg/day (Jankovic et al. 1984). Additional controlled studies are necessary to resolve these reported differences in efficacy.

Metoclopramide

Metoclopramide is a selective D_2 receptor antagonist. We treated four patients with metoclopramide at a maximum dosage of 240 mg/day, but only one had an excellent response of 95% decrease of tics (A. K. Shapiro et al. 1988). A complete remission of symptoms is reported in a single patient treated with a dosage of 240 mg/day for 12 weeks, with a return of symptoms when the dosage was reduced to 120 mg/day (Desai et al. 1983). The potential efficacy of metoclopramide has important theoretical implications because of its exclusive D_2 blocking properties and should be further evaluated using higher dosages. Although adverse effects were minimal in our patient, parkinsonism, tardive dyskinesia, and acute dystonic reactions have been reported (Bateman et al. 1983; Grimes et al. 1982; Leopold 1984; Patel 1986; Pollera et al. 1984).

Tiapride

This medication, not available in the United States, is reported to have dopaminergic blocking action mainly on D_2 receptors. It is related to both sulpiride and metoclopramide, of which it is a derivative. Tiapride was reported as effective as haloperidol but with fewer adverse effects in an open study of 15 children at a dosage of 100 mg tid (Pasquier and Pouplard 1977) and in an adolescent treated initially with 300 mg intramuscularly and subsequently with 900 mg/day orally (Lipcsey 1983). Tiapride was reported as ineffective at a daily dosage of 5 mg/kg in 10 children (Eggers et al. 1983).

Clozapine

Clozapine, an atypical neuroleptic thought to preferentially block mesolimbic but not nigrostriatal dopamine receptors, is an effective antipsychotic drug with few extrapyramidal effects (Meltzer et al. 1989). Adverse effects of the drug, however, include drowsiness, marked somnolence, salivation, and leukopenia. We used this drug to treat seven patients in the 1970s; although none developed extrapyramidal effects, neither did any improve on up to 800 mg/day of clozapine (A. K. Shapiro et al. 1988). It is significant that six of the seven patients had a previous good response to haloperidol. Clozapine also was reported as ineffective in a double-blind, crossover study for 4–7 weeks using dosages between 8 and 10 mg/kg/day (Caine et al. 1979).

Alpha-methylparatyrosine

Alpha-methylparatyrosine, which inhibits tyrosine hydroxylase, the rate limiting enzyme in catecholamine synthesis, was administered to six TS patients at a maximum dosage of 3,000 mg/day (A. K. Shapiro et al. 1978). Tics improved in three patients, especially dystonic neck and trunk movements in two of the patients, but three patients did not improve. The major limitation of this medication is microscopic, needle-like crystals that appeared in the urine of four patients, and crystalluria associated with decreased creatine clearance (50–60 ml/minute) in two patients. In addition, akinesia, akathisia, lethargy, and enuresis were sufficiently pronounced to nullify therapeutic effects. We also used a combination of alpha-methylparatyrosine and resperine in one patient without effect.

Piquindone

Piquindone, a D_2 receptor antagonist, was reported to be effective in an open clinical trial of three patients with TS and in a subsequent 1-month, double-blind, crossover study that included three patients who participated in the initial open trial (Uhr et al. 1984, 1986). Dosage varied from 20 to 50 mg/day. There was a moderate to marked reduction in motor tics and mild reduction of vocal tics. The only adverse effect was mild sedation. Unfortunately, clinical trials by the drug company have been terminated because of long-term toxic effects in animals.

Disulfiram

Disulfiram inhibits the enzyme dopamine-beta-hydroxylase, which catalyzes the conversion of dopamine to norepinephrine. Based on the theory that inhibition of dopamine-beta-hydroxylase should decrease the concentration of norepinephrine and enhance the accumulation of dopamine, two patients with TS were treated with disulfiram. Disulfiram at 1.5 mg/day had no effect on tics (A. K. Shapiro et al. 1978).

Ineffective and Controversial Treatments

A detailed review of many other drugs that have been tried in TS is reported in A. K. Shapiro et al. (1988). Almost all are clinically ineffective; a few have slight but limited usefulness or their use is controversial.

Ineffective Treatments

Ineffective drugs include dopamine agonists (such as apomorphine, pribedil, and levodopa), serotonin agonists (such as L-5-hydroxytryptophan and L-tryptophan), cholinergic agonists and antagonists (such as physostigmine, deanol, choline, lecithin, and benztropine mesylate), antidepressants (such as imipramine, amitriptyline, chlorimipramine, desipramine, monoamine oxidase inhibitors, lithium, and fluoxetine), anticonvulsants (such as carbamazepine, phenytoin, ethosuximide, primidone, and valproic acid), antianxiety–sedative-hypnotics (such as diazepam, chlordiazepoxide, flurazepam, and clorazepate), beta-blockers, corticosteroids, calcium-channel blockers (such as verapamil, diltiazem, and nifedipine), aminobutyric acid inhibitors (such as baclofen), allergic desensitization, megavitamins, and orthomolecular mineral therapy. Other ineffective treatment includes diet and nutrition, holistic treatment, electroconvulsive therapy, and insulin coma therapy. Several reports describe various central nervous system surgical treatments as effective, but severe organic adverse effects limit their use.

Controversial Treatments

Although clonidine has been extensively used for the treatment of TS, the data supporting its effectiveness are controversial. In an open crossover comparison of clonidine and neuroleptics, significantly more patients treated with neuroleptics (68.7%) improved compared with clonidine (13.5%) ($P < .0001$) (A. K. Shapiro et al. 1983b). The effectiveness of treatment with clonidine compared with placebo in 30 patients treated for 12 weeks in a double-blind study was not significantly different (Goetz et al. 1987). A limitation of this latter study is that prestudy neuroleptics were continued in 11 patients during the study. Although clonidine was reported significantly superior to placebo in a double-blind comparison of 40 patients treated for 12 weeks, the results were not significant when adjusted for the number of comparisons (Leckman et al. 1991). Goetz et al. concluded that clonidine is effective but less so than haloperidol and pimozide. Although some patients may benefit from clonidine, and it has few adverse effects, frequently it is effective only at dosages that cause sedation.

Clonazepam has been sporadically reported as effective in clinical reports (A. K. Shapiro et al. 1988; Troung et al. 1988). Its use is limited because of sedation and the development of tolerance similar to other benzodiazepines. Many patients previously treated with clonazepam did not improve, nor did patients treated by us, except for occasional patients whose symptoms retrospectively were different from patients with classical tics, such as those with a form of sensory tics and those who developed "fog states" or paranoia on neuroleptics (A. K. Shapiro et al. 1988).

Several initial clinical reports described naltrexone, an opiate antagonist (Kurlan et al. 1991; A. K. Shapiro et al. 1988), and nicotine potentiation of haloperidol (McConville et al. 1991) as potentially useful in TS. Botulinum serum injections, demonstrably effective in blepharospasm and other focal dystonic disorders, is a promising treatment for suppressing focal tics such as eye blinking and warrants further evaluation.

Psychotherapy, psychoanalysis, hypnosis, and other psychological therapy are not effective treatments for tic disorders and TS. Various behavioral techniques have been extensively reported as effective, but the studies usually describe single patients and do not utilize control groups, specific diagnostic criteria, standardized outcome measures, double-blind procedures, evidence of generalization, and follow-up evaluation (A. K. Shapiro et al. 1978, 1988). An exception to these shortcomings is a study utilizing habit reversal in 10 patients treated in 13–30 sessions over 8–11 months who were compared with a waiting list control group; there was a 93% reduction of tics reported (Azrin and Peterson 1990). Targeted behavioral techniques for discrete or focal symptoms, especially for recalcitrant symptoms such as coprolalia or spitting, might be effective and warrant further evaluation.

Evaluation of Efficacy Complicated by Spontaneous, Nonspecific, and Placebo Effects

The difficulty of evaluating the effectiveness of treatment for tics and TS is complicated by spontaneous waxing, waning, and fluctuation of symptoms and nonspecific or placebo effects. In our sample of 666 TS patients (A. K. Shapiro et al. 1988), 97% had a spontaneous change in the severity of symptoms (waxing and waning of symptoms), 96% a spontaneous change in the type of symptoms (fluctuation of symptoms), and 27% a spontaneous remission lasting from 2 weeks to 7 years. Other factors contributing to changes in the severity of symptoms are diurnal variation, seasonal factors, situational stimuli, and other possible nonspecific or placebo effects. In fact, the magnitude of these spontaneous changes often exceeds the percentage of improvement reported in many uncontrolled clinical studies. Moreover, waxing, waning, and fluctuation of symptoms are criteria for all tic disorders in DSM-III-R.

This problem can be illustrated by a retrospective analysis of the effect of placebo in one of our studies (A. K. Shapiro and Shapiro 1984). For 20 patients treated with placebo for 6 weeks, tics increased, decreased, or were unchanged in about one-third of patients, respectively. Similar results were apparent in a subsequent controlled crossover study of 57 patients treated with haloperidol, pimozide, and placebo (E. Shapiro et al. 1989). These results suggest that nonplacebo effects should exceed improvement in more than one-third of treated TS patients. However, the range for improvement on placebo varies from 10% to 55% with different dependent variables. Change, therefore, may be related more to the type of dependent variable used in the study than to the effect of the treatment. Even worse is the tendency to select one of many dependent improvement variables retrospectively, usually based on which variable shows the most improvement.

Another important consideration in determining spontaneous and placebo effects includes the patients' expectations that the new medication will result in symptomatic improvement. In addition, patients generally seek treatment or a change to a new medication when they are at their worst, thus maximizing subsequent improvement with any treatment because of the likelihood of spontaneous improvement. Also, if an active drug that has adverse effects is discontinued at the height of an illness, and a new drug is administered just before the onset of spontaneous waning of symptoms, improvement and decreased adverse effects are likely to be attributed to the newly administered drug. These factors underscore the necessity of conducting well-controlled, hypothesis-oriented, double-blind studies that include dependent improvement measures with evidence of reliability and validity to evaluate the efficacy of treatment in TS.

Predictors of Improvement

To evaluate possible predictors of improvement associated with treatment with haloperidol or pimozide, independent variables and dependent improvement variables at endpoint were retrospectively examined in several studies (A. K. Shapiro and Shapiro 1984; A. K. Shapiro et al. 1978, 1988; E. Shapiro et al. 1989). Independent variables included age, sex, history of tics or TS, age at onset of TS, severity of TS, diagnosis of attention-deficit disorder with and without hyperactivity, Conners Abbreviated Parental

Scale (Hyperactivity Index), severity of behavioral symptoms (hyperactivity, obsessive-compulsive symptoms, compulsive personality, anger-mood, inhibition, learning disorders, coordination abilities, and intellectual-psychosocial functioning), dosage of haloperidol or pimozide, use of benztropine mesylate, previously untreated or treated with medication, type of neuroleptic (haloperidol, pimozide, or fluphenazine), and previous response to treatment. The dependent variables included the TS Severity Scale and the Clinical Global Impression Scale. None of the correlations was significant except for negative correlations of age with ratings of improvement on the Clinical Global Impression Scale (haloperidol, $r = -0.56$, $P = .003$; pimozide, $r = -0.39$, $P = .04$). However, these results are within chance expectations because 52 correlations were examined. Response to treatment, therefore, cannot be predicted at this time.

The effectiveness of dopamine blocking neuroleptics, particularly those with predominant D_2 blocking effects, is the major empirical finding implicating, but not proving, dopamine as having an etiological relationship to TS. Evaluation of efficacy is complicated by spontaneous, nonspecific, and placebo effects and underscores the limitations of uncontrolled studies and the need to conduct methodologically rigorous studies to evaluate the effectiveness of drug treatment for tics and TS.

The reviewed evidence provides more support for the overall effectiveness and known patterns of adverse effects for haloperidol, pimozide, and fluphenazine than for other neuroleptics and all other drug categories. The discussion of the clinical treatment of tics and TS, therefore, focuses on these drugs.

General Considerations About Treatment of Tic Disorders

Indications for Treatment

In our opinion, the guiding principle of clinical practice should be that transient tic disorder, chronic motor or vocal tic disorder, and TS have a similar undetermined organic central nervous system etiology and that treatment should be directed primarily at reducing tic symptoms. Pharmacological treatment is indicated if the symptoms markedly impair psychosocial, educational, or occupational functioning. Because treatment is palliative, treatment is unnecessary if the symptoms are very mild, do not elicit comment and curiosity by outside observers, and do not interfere with psychosocial functioning. Treatment of mild symptoms is elective and should be determined by the patient and family based on the degree of distress caused by the tics. Moderately severe symptoms usually require treatment; very severe symptoms always require treatment. In addition, psychotherapy may be indicated for some patients who are overly sensitive to the presence of very mild tics, for those who have an excessive psychological reaction to their tics, or those who have another disorder requiring treatment.

Clinical Course and Prognosis

An important consideration underlying treatment is the natural course and prognosis for tic disorders (A. K. Shapiro et al. 1988). The clinical course is variable, characterized by spontaneous waxing, waning, or fluctuation of symptoms over time. Complete remission, usually before adolescence, occurs in about 9% of patients; periodic remissions last 2 weeks to 7 years in about 30% of patients; and, in the remainder, a chronic lifelong course is evident. Although the severity of symptoms over time cannot be predicted in individual patients, the severity of tics decreases in about 30% of patients during adolescence and in most patients in adulthood. Some patients have severe brief or prolonged exacerbations sometime in adulthood. Symptoms are usually decreased by absorption in tasks, in the presence of strangers, and outside the home and are usually increased while at home with family or close friends and when aroused. The symptoms are usually less severe in the morning, increase in the afternoon, and are maximum in the evening.

General Principles of Treatment With Neuroleptics

An important principle of treatment with neuroleptics for both children and adults is that the dosage—influenced by level of liver enzymes and genetic, metabolic, and pharmacokinetic factors—has to be individually titrated to achieve maximum effectiveness with minimal adverse effects. Dosage for children, largely similar to adults, except for lower dosage for young children, is determined by pragmatic clinical trial and error (Geller 1991). Functioning TS patients report more bothersome and impairing adverse effects with lower dosages of neuroleptics than are commonly reported by psychotic patients who are treated with much higher dosages. Unfortunately, blood levels of medication used at therapeutically appropriate dosages are not useful because they are not correlated with age, weight, sex, severity, clinical response, or adverse effects (Geller 1991). Neuroleptics have a long half-life and tend to accumulate in the body so that the same dosage over time results in higher cumulative blood levels. A steady blood level state is reached in about 4 days. Thus the clinical effect should be evaluated after 4–7 days during initial titration, and the dosage should be changed appropriately on the fifth to seventh day. The elimination of the drug takes about 4 days during initial acute treatment and ranges from 4 to 30 days, usually averaging 2 weeks, with chronic treatment. On withdrawal, adverse effects tend to decrease and disappear before the tics reappear at their preexisting level. Because neuroleptics have a long half-life, the total dosage can be administered at bedtime for most patients. Akinesic or sedative effects may increase after intake and are often better tolerated by patients during sleep. Once-a-day, nighttime administration contributes to ease of administration and improves compliance, although some patients have a better response and fewer adverse effects if medication is administered at intervals throughout the day.

Treatment Regimen

Haloperidol, Fluphenazine, and Pimozide

Although treatment of tic disorders with neuroleptics is largely similar to treatment of psychoses, nonpsychiatrically impaired individuals with tic disorders are more sensitive to adverse effects. The treatment regimen therefore requires modification. We recommend that the starting dosage for most children and adults be low, such as 0.25 mg/day of haloperidol and fluphenazine or 1.0 mg of pimozide. (Equivalent dosages of chlorpromazine are 12.5 mg, 12.5 mg, and 33.3 mg, respectively.) Such small doses present some problems in administration because these medications come in predetermined dosages. The smallest dosage forms are 0.5-mg scored tablets for haloperidol (one half tablet every day yielding an average daily dose of 0.25 mg), 1-mg unscored tablets for fluphenazine (one tablet every fourth day yielding an average daily dosage of 0.25 mg), and 2.0-mg scored tablets for pimozide (one half tablet every day yielding an average daily dosage of 1.0 mg). As has been mentioned previously, medication is best administered at bedtime. To prevent acute dystonia, which occurs in 5%–9% of patients usually within 72 hours, and acute akinesia, which occurs in 25% of patients usually within the first 2 weeks of treatment, the anticholinergic drug, benztropine mesylate, at a dosage of 0.5 mg at bedtime, can be used routinely at the beginning of treatment.

Dosage of haloperidol and fluphenazine is increased 0.25 mg every 5–7 days and pimozide, 1 mg every 5–7 days until either symptoms decrease substantially without adverse effects, adverse effects occur without symptomatic benefit, or symptoms decrease and adverse effects occur at the same time. The latter possibility is the usual response. If adverse effects are minimal and do not interfere with functioning, such as slightly increased sedation at bedtime and on awakening, dosage should not be increased until these adverse effects disappear. If adverse effects interfere slightly with functioning, dosage should be decreased by the same amount per week. If adverse effects are severe, dosage should be reduced 50% immediately. Titration should be reinstituted more slowly at intervals varying between 7 and 30 days after disappearance of severe adverse effects. More rapid titration, 0.25–1 mg every day or even every hour, is feasible in patients with very severe TS. Although the dosage ranges from 1.5 to 10 mg/day for haloperidol, 1.5 to 30 mg/day for pimozide, and 2 to 15 mg/day for fluphenazine, higher doses are required by some patients. Effective dosages are unrelated to weight, age, sex, and other relative variables, although the range for children tends to be lower than for adults (A. K. Shapiro et al. 1988).

The goal of treatment is to reduce tics at least 70% in school, at work, with strangers, and in social situations. Symptoms are usually more severe at home, in the evening; although it is possible to control symptoms at home by increasing the dosage, to do so usually results in increased adverse effects. Symptom reduction can be as high as 90%–99% without adverse effects in some patients, although others achieve only 50%–60% reduction of tics. Because symptoms vary spontaneously, continued flexible titration of dosage is recommended so that patients are on the lowest possible dosage and have minimal adverse effects. Moreover, titrating the dosage over time allows the physician to detect spontaneous decrease or remission of symptoms.

Penfluridol

Penfluridol has a longer half-life than haloperidol and differs in dosage ratio and frequency of administration. Penfluridol is administered daily or once every 3–7 days, at an initial dose of 10 mg. Dosage is increased usually in 10-mg increments every 3–7 days to the point of maximum benefit and minimal adverse effects. At that point, the total dosage for the preceding week can be given weekly or in divided doses during the week. After chronic use, dosage can be given at intervals of 1–4 weeks. The median weekly dosage is about 40 mg, with a range of 20–140 mg. Adverse effects disappear and clinical symptoms return 1–6 weeks after penfluridol is withdrawn because of its long half-life. Adverse effects are similar to those of haloperidol except for less severe akinesia. Management of adverse effects should follow those outlined for haloperidol.

Laboratory Testing

Jaundice and agranulocytosis occur infrequently, especially with the use of haloperidol, pimozide, and fluphenazine. The time frame for neuroleptic-induced jaundice is in the first 5 weeks of treatment and for agranulocytosis, the 4th to 10th week of treatment. Prodromal symptoms for hepatitis include malaise, fever, and flu-like symptoms, which may develop into a yellow color of the sclera and skin. Laboratory tests for hepatitis might include bilirubin, SGPT (serum glutamic-pyruvic transaminase), SGOT (serum glutamic-oxaloacetic transaminase), and alkaline phosphatase. The jaundice is usually benign, and patients recover whether or not the medication is continued. Agranulocytosis cannot be anticipated by serial blood counts and is usually diagnosed by the sudden appearance of a high fever and an overwhelming infection, usually oral or pharyngeal, caused by a precipitous drop in the white blood count. It is important to stop medication immediately because the mortality increases to 40% with continued use. Most experienced clinicians do not recommend weekly or routine blood determinations but use them only with the appearance of the clinical symptoms suggesting or associated with these adverse effects. If agranulocytosis is suspected, a white blood and differential count should be obtained.

A statement in the *Physicians' Desk Reference*, prompted by the FDA, cautions that pimozide not be the first drug used to treat TS patients, that its use should be limited to severely afflicted patients who fail to respond to standard medication, that dosages greater than 10 mg/day or 0.2 mg/kg are not recommended, and that patients be required to have initial and periodic electrocardiograms (ECGs) during dosage titration. The dosage ratio is estimated as 2–4 mg of pimozide to 1 mg of haloperidol.

These recommendations are based on two sudden deaths, possibly due to cardiac arrest, that were reported in a national collaborative study of pimozide in acute schizophrenic patients whose dosage was increased to 80 mg in 2 weeks (Fulop et al. 1987). In our double-blind, crossover study of 57 patients treated for 6 weeks with pimozide, haloperidol, and placebo, clinically significant cardiac effects did not occur at a maximum dosage of 0.3 mg/kg or 20 mg/day for pimozide and 10 mg/day for haloperidol (A. K. Shapiro et al. 1987; E. Shapiro et al. 1989). However, the QTc interval was significantly prolonged during treatment with pimozide compared with haloperidol, although values for both medications were not in an abnormal range. The differential effect on the QTc interval may be related to the fact that pimozide and other diphenylbutylpiperidines, in contrast to butyrophenones, have calcium-channel blocking properties. Impeding the influx of calcium delays cardiac repolarization, thereby increasing the QTc interval. The increase in the QTc interval was always within 25% of baseline values and occurred within 3 weeks of starting treatment.

These preliminary results indicate that periodic ECG monitoring may be unnecessary for TS patients without histories of cardiac disease or prolonged QTc intervals, and if the dose is titrated gradually to maximum dosage. Erenberg (1988) reported that serial ECGs in children treated with pimozide revealed no significant alteration in QT intervals. He noted that he no longer performs routine follow-up ECGs. However, further study of all neuroleptics is warranted, using 24-hour ECG monitoring and especially after glucose loads, which are associated with T wave changes during neuroleptic treatment (Chouinard and Annable 1977).

Because an ECG at baseline and unspecified subsequent ECGs are recommended in the *Physicians' Desk Reference,* some clinicians may opt to monitor treatment with ECGs. The following conservative guidelines are suggested: Patients with QTc intervals above 0.44 seconds should not be treated except after approval by a cardiac consultant. If T wave alteration (except T wave inversion) occurs, the dose should not be increased, ECGs should be repeated, and the patient closely observed. If during treatment the QTc interval exceeds 25% of baseline or 0.47 seconds in children and 0.52 seconds in adults, or if other T wave alterations occur, the dose should be reduced until repeated ECGs are normal. If U wave or T wave inversion is observed, or cardiac arrhythmia develops, pimozide should be discontinued, and ECGs should be repeated until normal. If bradycardia (less than 50 beats per minute) occurs, the dose should be reduced until the pulse is normal. The recommendations for the use of pimozide otherwise are similar to those outlined for haloperidol except for the dosage ratio of 2–4 mg of pimozide to 1 mg of haloperidol.

Treatment of Comorbid Disorders

Use of Stimulants in Treating ADHD

The association of ADHD with TS and its treatment with stimulants are controversial. ADHD is thought to be genetically associated with TS by Comings and Comings (1984), to occur more frequently than expected but not genetically associated with TS by Pauls et al. (1986), and unassociated with TS but reported more frequently than expected because of ascertainment bias by A. K. Shapiro et al. (1988). Also controversial is whether the use of stimulants is indicated (Comings and Comings 1984; A. K. Shapiro and Shapiro 1981; A. K. Shapiro et al. 1988; Sverd et al. 1989) or contraindicated (Golden 1974; Lowe et al. 1982) for the treatment of ADHD associated with TS or in patients with a history of tics in the family. The controversy and the rationale for the use of stimulants to treat ADHD and to counteract the adverse effects of neuroleptic-induced adverse effects are discussed comprehensively elsewhere (A. K. Shapiro et al. 1988).

Some authors, based on retrospective reports, have concluded that stimulants can cause tics, worsen or permanently exacerbate tics, or precipitate TS (Golden 1977a; Lowe et al. 1982). Others have concluded that high dosages of stimulants may cause a temporary increase in tics but that stimulants do not precipitate or permanently worsen TS. In fact, stimulants may decrease tics, especially in children with hyperactivity, who may require a trial on stimulants if hyperactivity and attentional problems are severe. In our opinion, there is inadequate evidence that stimulants precipitate or permanently exacerbate TS. This conclusion is supported by a study of patients with ADHD who later developed TS (Comings and Comings 1984). The authors reasoned that if stimulants were associated with the development of TS, ADHD patients treated with stimulants should develop TS earlier than patients who were not treated with stimulants. They found, however, that ADHD patients treated with stimulants developed TS at a significantly later age than patients not treated with stimulants.

Further support for the lack of association between stimulant use and subsequent TS is provided in a study of six identical twins with ADHD in which one twin, but not the other, was treated with stimulants (Price et al. 1986). Both twins developed TS whether they were pretreated with stimulants or not. Additional support for the use of stimulants in patients with ADHD and TS is found in the study by Sverd et al. (1989).

Stimulants may increase, have no effect on, or decrease tics in about one-third of patients respectively (A. K. Shapiro et al. 1988). Similar observations have been made by others (Butler 1985; Comings and Comings 1984; Erenberg et al. 1985; Sverd et al. 1989). Although tics may increase in susceptible patients, especially if higher dosages are used, the increase is short-lived and the potential benefits of stimulants often outweigh their disadvantages. Many patients have been successfully treated with a combination of a neuroleptic and stimulant, and we and others consider stimulants to be necessary agents for the treatment and management of children with TS and clinically significant hyperactivity (Comings and Comings 1984; Konkol et al. 1990; A. K. Shapiro and Shapiro 1981; Sverd et al. 1989).

Clinical Use of Stimulants

The decision about whether to treat patients with both ADHD and TS initially with neuroleptics or stimulants is based on which disorder interferes most with psychosocial functioning. If both require treatment, we usually treat TS first, as outlined previously, and ADHD subsequently. Initial treatment if indicated should titrate the stimulant slowly to an appropriate dosage that minimizes ADHD symptoms and does not cause adverse effects (Elia 1991). Methylphenidate is given at an initial dosage of 2.5 mg on awakening and subsequently titrated in daily increments of 2.5 mg/day, in divided dosages, to a dosage of 0.3 mg/kg/day to 1.0 mg/kg/day or in a dosage range of 5–80 mg/day. The results are often dramatic. If tics increase, they readily subside within 6 hours after reduction of dosage.

Other stimulants, such as dextroamphetamine (5–40 mg/day), sustained-release methamphetamine or dextroamphetamine, and magnesium pemoline, can also be used. Pemoline, a long-lasting stimulant, can be administered once daily and titrated up or down at weekly intervals, the dosage varying between 18.75 and 150 mg/day. An advantage of pemoline is its sustained effect throughout the day without the acute "rush" effect of methylphenidate, which is experienced as dysphoric by some patients. The use of pemoline is limited, however, because periodic liver function tests are required to detect hepatotoxicity estimated to occur in 2% of patients treated for about 10–12 months (Nehra 1990).

Alternative drugs that are more effective than placebo but probably less effective than stimulants and that do not increase tics include imipramine and desipramine, which are slowly titrated to 75–125 mg/day. However, the use of desipramine is limited because of recent reports of cardiac fatalities; such reports indicate that use of desipramine requires careful monitoring with ECGs. Similar adverse effects have not been reported for imipramine. Similarly, clonidine, at a daily dosage of 0.05 mg, is administered once per day for 1 week; increased to twice a day for 1 week, three times a day for 1 week, and so on; and increased

0.05 mg each week, to a maximum of 0.1 mg every three or four times per day. Behavioral techniques specifically targeted at learning and psychosocial problems are generally helpful when indicated. If tics spontaneously increase, or if stimulants are associated with increased tics (usually only slightly), then treatment with neuroleptics, as previously described, may be indicated.

Comprehensive neuropsychological testing by experienced psychologists is often necessary and helpful to differentiate ADHD from conduct disorder, other psychopathology, and diverse organic disorders. Finally, as of this writing, we are aware of six filed malpractice suits in the United States, but only one, for $1.4 million, was brought—unsuccessfully—to trial. For these and other reasons, including warnings about tardive dyskinesia from neuroleptics, which is exceedingly infrequent in TS patients (A. K. Shapiro et al. 1988), obtaining an appropriate signed consent is obligatory.

Behavioral Problems, Psychopathology, and OCS-OCD

The controversy about whether behavioral problems, ADHD, OCS-OCD, and diverse psychopathology, from mild anxiety to schizophrenia, are etiologically related to the onset of TS or are comorbid features associated with TS is comprehensively evaluated elsewhere (A. K. Shapiro and Shapiro 1992; A. K. Shapiro et al. 1988). Papers in the literature proposing a relationship between these psychopathological states and tic disorders include anecdotal and uncontrolled clinical reports or opinions and very few inadequately controlled retrospective studies. Our clinical experience and controlled predictive studies indicate that TS patients without attention-deficit disorder do not differ significantly from a carefully matched control group without TS on measures of psychopathology, whereas TS patients with attention-deficit disorder have significantly more psychopathology than TS patients without attention-deficit disorder and a control group without TS, and are similar to a sample of patients referred to mental health facilities (A. K. Shapiro et al. 1988). Similarly, a comprehensive review of the literature concluded that the evidence does not support the conclusion that OCS-OCD is associated with tic disorders (A. K. Shapiro and Shapiro 1992; A. K. Shapiro et al. 1988).

Our conclusion is that the frequency of behavior problems, psychopathology, attention-deficit disorder, and OCS-OCD is no greater among patients with tic disorders than in the general population. Adequate but currently unavailable controlled studies are required to confirm these hypotheses. The controversy and limitations of the evidence are acknowledged in DSM-III-R: "In clinical samples, other mental disorders are frequently associated with Tourette's Disorder, particularly attention-deficit hyperactivity disorder and obsessive compulsive disorder. It is not clear if this co-morbidity also exists in representative community samples" (American Psychiatric Association 1987, p. 79).

Whether confirmed or not, the treatment of potential comorbid disorders requires treatment other than use of neuroleptics for TS. For example, although neuroleptics are effective for the treatment of tic disorders, they are not effective for the treatment of ADHD, OCS-OCD, and many other possible disorders. Patients with concurrent OCS-OCD are not helped by neuroleptic drugs but may be helped by antiobsessional drugs, which do not benefit tics. Similar parallels occur for concurrent ADHD, various behavioral problems, psychopathology, and physical illnesses.

Recognition and Management of Adverse Effects

Most psychiatrists are familiar with the recognition and management of neuroleptic-induced adverse effects in psychiatrically ill patients, but usually not in patients with TS who are otherwise normal. Certain adverse effects may be more difficult to detect in patients with florid psychiatric symptoms for which neuroleptics are used and only become apparent during remissions. Moreover, otherwise-normal individuals with TS may be more sensitive to lower dosages, which can seriously interfere with functioning. In this section, we describe adverse effects encountered in patients with TS that are often misidentified or mismanaged. A comprehensive discussion of adverse effects appears elsewhere (A. K. Shapiro et al. 1988).

Both clinical response and adverse effects associated with haloperidol, pimozide, and fluphenazine are essentially similar.

Although the discussion of adverse effects focuses on the treatment of tic disorders with haloperidol, these adverse effects occur with pimozide, fluphenazine, penfluridol, and other neuroleptics.

Cognitive Impairment

Cognitive impairment is a subtle and major limitation of the use of neuroleptics. It appears to be an akinesic or tranquilizing effect that impairs sustained attention and interferes with motivation, memory, and performance, although the precise modality of the impairment is unknown. Parents report a decline in school grades, and both children and adults experience a decrease in work performance and motivation. Although cognitive impairment appears to be dose related, it may occur at very low dosages in susceptible individuals, such as 1.5 mg/day of haloperidol (75 mg CPZ-EQ). Management requires constant titration to the minimal dosage required for maximum improvement outside the home, a trial on anticholinergics (which are rarely effective), or the use of stimulants (which are usually effective).

Dysphoria, Irritability, and Depressive and Phobic Adverse Effects

These adverse effects are also related to dosage and may occur at very low doses in susceptible individuals. These drug-induced adverse effects are similar to those occurring in patients treated with reserpine for hypertension. Patients frequently complain of dysphoria in various ways: sadness, crying spells, depression, and occasional suicidal thoughts (Bruun 1982; Caine and Polinsky 1979; A. K. Shapiro et al. 1978, 1988). Premorbid characteristics that predispose patients to the development of depression have not yet been identified. Children express these adverse effects most frequently as irritability, similar to that of a tired child, and parents report personality changes in their children. Anticholinergics, antidepressants, and psychotherapy are usually not effective in controlling these adverse effects. Although tolerance may develop over time, management usually requires decreasing the dosage of the neuroleptic or introducing the use of stimulants, which very effectively control these adverse effects. Symptoms of separation anxiety and phobias, which may occur in children on low dosages (Linet 1985; Mikkelsen et al. 1981; A. K. Shapiro and Shapiro 1980;

A. K. Shapiro et al. 1988), have been treated effectively with tricyclic antidepressants.

Management of Neuroleptic-Induced Adverse Effects With Stimulants

Stimulants are also routinely used by us to control intractable neuroleptic-induced adverse effects of akinesia; sedation; lethargy; dysphoria; depression; cognitive and motivational blunting; and impaired academic, occupational, and psychosocial functioning. Although tics occasionally increase slightly in susceptible patients, especially when stimulants are administered at higher dosages, the increase is short-lived and readily decreases with dosage reduction; the potential benefits of stimulants outweigh presumed disadvantages. Another effect is decreased appetite and loss of weight.

A major principle of treatment with stimulants is constant, sensitive, and subtle titration of the dosage so that maximum relief of symptoms can be achieved with minimal discomfort from adverse effects. Similar beneficial effects of stimulants have been reported for schizophrenic patients who were impaired psychosocially by the akinesic effects of neuroleptics (Ayd 1964).

"Fog States"

"Fog states," characterized by feelings of depersonalization, paranoia, and slowed mentation, lasting from a few seconds to several hours, not present before the use or after discontinuation of neuroleptics, were experienced by several patients on moderate dosages of neuroleptics (A. K. Shapiro et al. 1988). Two of the patients had fog states when on more than 15 mg/day of haloperidol. One patient developed rushing thoughts, paranoia, adversive head movements to either side, and frequent tics after 3 years of haloperidol therapy. He also reported many episodes of having his thoughts repetitively fixate on a part of his body, an object, or a word. A second patient had repetitive psychopathological fantasies. A psychological cause for these fantasies was not obvious. Their presence would ordinarily indicate severe psychopathology, but the patient was neither psychotic nor obsessive-compulsive. If these symptoms occur, especially in the presence of a subtle, organic mental syndrome, the dosage should be reduced, or trial periods on and off medication should be undertaken to evaluate whether medication is the cause of the fog state. The exact extent and relationship of these fog states and fixated ideas to neuroleptics and TS are unclear. Their existence needs to be further documented and studied.

Paranoid States

Some adults as well as children with TS receiving low dosages of haloperidol or pimozide have experienced brief paranoid states, although these states occur infrequently. Such reactions have not been observed in schizophrenic patients on neuroleptics. There is as yet no explanation for these atypical side effects, whose characteristics appear to be different clinically from the paranoid symptoms seen in general psychiatric patients.

Conclusion

The foregoing discussion has demonstrated that the proper treatment of tics or TS symptoms is suppression of the tics with medication if they interfere with the child's psychosocial functioning. Neuroleptics such as haloperidol, pimozide, and fluphenazine are the most effective drugs for the treatment of tics and TS. Clinical experience with these medications indicates that patients who fail to improve on one medication may be helped by another. The pattern of effectiveness, adverse effects, and management strategies are essentially similar for all neuroleptics except for dosages. Although there is now a wider choice of medications to treat patients with tic disorders than in the past, more effective medications, with fewer adverse effects and greater ease of use by nonspecialists, are still needed.

Well-designed studies are necessary to clarify further the efficacy and limitations of current and future treatment of tic disorders. These studies should incorporate accepted methodological principles such as blind evaluation of patients and control subjects to avoid observer bias, the use of clinical samples rather than volunteers to avoid ascertainment bias (P. Cohen and Cohen 1984), the use of an appropriate control group to control for social desirability, random assignment to treatments, stringent criteria for defining tic disorders, a priori specification of hypotheses, independent and dependent variables and statistical procedures, adequate sample size, the use of test instruments with demonstrated reliability and validity to control for errors in measurement, and, finally, the appropriate adjustment of the significance level in retrospective analyses to avoid overidentifying cases as positive (i.e., making Type 1 errors) (Yusuf et al. 1991). Because such studies are not easy to conduct, especially because large clinical samples are difficult for individual investigators to obtain, collaborative studies may be necessary to optimize the understanding of TS and its pharmacological treatment in children.

References

American Psychiatric Association: Diagnostic and Statistical Manual of Mental Disorders, 3rd Edition, Revised. Washington, DC, American Psychiatric Association, 1987

American Psychiatric Association: Diagnostic and Statistical Manual of Mental Disorders, 4th Edition. Washington, DC, American Psychiatric Association, 1994

Anden NE, Butcher SG, Corrodi H, et al: Receptor activity and turnover of dopamine and noradrenaline after neuroleptics. Eur J Pharmacol 11:303–314, 1970

Ayd FJ: Protracted administration of methylphenidate (Ritalin). Psychosomatics 5:180–187, 1964

Azrin NH, Peterson AL: Treatment of Tourette syndrome by habit reversal: a waiting-list control group comparison. Behavior Therapy 21:305–318, 1990

Bateman DN, Craft AW, Nicholson E, et al: Dystonic reactions and the pharmacokinetics of metoclopramide in children. Br J Clin Pharmacol 15:557–559, 1983

Borison RL, Ang L, Chang S: New pharmacological approaches in the treatment of Tourette syndrome, in Advances in Neurology, Vol 35, Gilles de la Tourette Syndrome. Edited by Friedhoff AJ, Chase TN. New York, Raven, 1982, pp 377–382

Boswell J: The Life of Samuel Johnson. London, Everyman, 1791

Bruun RD: Dysphoric phenomena associated with haloperidol treatment of Tourette syndrome, in Advances in Neurology, Vol 35, Gilles de la Tourette Syndrome. Edited by Friedhoff AJ, Chase TN. New York, Raven, 1982, pp 433–436

Butler M: Review of developmental-behavioral pediatrics. Am J Psychiatry 142:876–877, 1985

Caine ED, Polinsky RJ: Haloperidol induced dysphoria in patients with Tourette syndrome. Am J Psychiatry 136:1216–1217, 1979

Caine ED, Polinsky RJ, Kartzinel R, et al: The trial use of clozapine for abnormal involuntary movement disorders. Am J Psychiatry 136:317–320, 1979

Caprini G, Melotti V: Un grave sindrome ticcosa guarita con haloperidol. Rivista Sperimentale Frenait 85:191–196, 1961

Casamenti F, Bianchi C, Beani L, et al: Effect of haloperidol and pimozide on acetylcholine output from the cerebral cortex in rats and guinea pigs. Eur J Pharmacol 65:279–284, 1980

Chouinard G, Annable L: Phenothiazine-induced ECG abnormalities. Arch Gen Psychiatry 34:951–954, 1977

Cohen DJ, Detlor J, Young JG, et al: Clonidine ameliorates Gilles de la Tourette syndrome. Arch Gen Psychiatry 37:1350–1357, 1980

Cohen P, Cohen J: The clinician's illusion. Arch Gen Psychiatry 41:1178–1182, 1984

Comings DE, Comings BG: Tourette syndrome and attention deficit disorder with hyperactivity: are they due to the same gene? Journal of the American Academy of Child Psychiatry 23:138–146 1984

Debray P, Messerschmitt PL, Lonchap D, et al: L'utilization du pimozide en pedopsychiatrie. La Nouvelle Presse Médicale 1:2917–2918, 1972

Desai AB, Doongaji DR, Satoskar RS: Metoclopramide in Gilles de la Tourette's syndrome (a case report). J Postgrad Med 29:181–183, 1983

Eggers C, Olbricht T, Rotherberger A: Neurobiological findings in children with tics and Gilles de la Tourette syndrome, in Special Aspects of Psychopharmacology. Edited by Ackenheil M, Matussek N. Paris, France, Expansion Scientifique Francaise, 1983, pp 191–202

Elia J: Stimulants and antidepressant pharmacokinetics in hyperactive children. Psychopharmacol Bull 27:411–415, 1991

Erenberg G: Pharmacologic therapy of tics in childhood. Pediatr Ann 17:1–7, 1988

Erenberg G, Cruse RP, Rothner D: Gilles de la Tourette syndrome: effects of stimulant drugs. Neurology 35:1346–1348, 1985

Fernando SJM: Gilles de la Tourette's syndrome. Br J Psychiatry 113:607–617, 1967

Ford CV, Gottlieb F: An objective evaluation of haloperidol in Gilles de la Tourette's syndrome. Diseases of the Nervous System 30:328–332, 1969

Fulop G, Phillips RA, Shapiro AK, et al: ECG changes during haloperidol and pimozide treatment of Tourette's disorder. Am J Psychiatry 144:673–675, 1987

Geller B: Psychopharmacology of children and adolescents: pharmacokinetics and relationships of plasma/serum levels to response. Psychopharmacol Bull 27:401–409, 1991

Gilles de la Tourette G: Etude sur une affection nerveuse caracterisee par de l'incoordination motrice accompagnee d'echolalie et de copralalie. Arch Neurol 9:19–42, 158–200, 1885

Goetz CG, Tanner CM, Klawans H: Fluphenazine and multifocal tic disorders. Arch Neurol 41:271–272, 1984

Goetz CG, Tanner CM, Wilson RS, et al: Clonidine and Gilles de la Tourette's syndrome: double-blind study using objective rating methods. Ann Neurol 21:307–310, 1987

Goldberg LI: Dopamine: receptors and clinical applications. Clin Physiol Biochem 3:120–126, 1985

Golden GS: Gilles de la Tourette's syndrome following methylphenidate administration. Dev Med Child Neurol 16:76–78, 1974

Golden GS: The effect of central nervous stimulants on Tourette syndrome. Ann Neurol 2:69–70, 1977a

Golden GS: The pediatric perspective. Am J Dis Child 131:531–534, 1977b

Grimes JD, Hassan MN, Preston DN: Adverse neurologic effects of metoclopramide. Can Med Assoc J 126:23–25, 1982

Holomboe R: Paper presented at the Sixth World Conference on Psychiatry, Honolulu, Hawaii, August 1977

Itard JMG: Memoire sur quelques fonctions involontaires des appareils de la locomotion de la prehension et de la voix. Archives Generale Médicine 8:385–407, 1825

Jankovic J, Glaze DG, Frost JD: Effect of tetrabenazine on tics and sleep of Gilles de la Tourette's syndrome. Neurology 34:688–692, 1984

Konkol RJ, Fischer M, Newby RF: Double blind, placebo-control stimulant trial in children with Tourette's syndrome and attention deficit hyperactive disorder. Annals of Neurobiology 28:424, 1990

Kramer H, Sprenger J: The Malleus Maleficarum (1489). Translated by Summers M. New York, Dover Publications, 1971

Kurlan R, Lichter D, Hewitt D: Sensory tics in Tourette's syndrome. Neurology 39:731–734, 1989

Kurlan R, Majumdar L, Deeley C, et al: A controlled trial of propoxyphene and naltrexone in patients with Tourette's syndrome. Ann Neurol 30:19–23, 1991

Leckman JF, Cohen DJ, Detlor J, et al: Clonidine in the treatment of Tourette syndrome: a review of data, in Advances in Neurology, Vol 35, Gilles de la Tourette Syndrome. Edited by Friedhoff AJ, Chase TN. New York, Raven, 1982, pp 391–401

Leckman JF, Hardin MT, Riddle MA, et al: Clonidine treatment of Gilles de la Tourette's syndrome. Arch Gen Psychiatry 48:324–328, 1991

Lees AJ: Tics and Related Disorders (Clinical Neurology and Neurosurgery Monographs, Vol 7). New York, Churchill Livingstone, 1985

Leopold NA: Prolonged metoclopramide-induced dyskinetic reaction. Neurology 34:238–239, 1984

Linet LS: Tourette syndrome, pimozide and school phobia: the neuroleptic separation anxiety syndrome. Am J Psychiatry 142:613–615, 1985

Lipcsey A: A propos de la maladie de Gilles de la Tourette. Semaine de Hopitaux de Paris 59:695–696, 1983

Lowe TL, Cohen DJ, Detlor J, et al: Stimulant medications precipitate Tourette's syndrome. JAMA 247:1168–1169, 1982

Matthysse S: Antipsychotic drug action: a clue to the neuropathology of schizophrenia? Federation Proceedings: Federation of American Societies for Experimental Biology (Bethesda) 32:200–205, 1973

McConville BJ, Fogelson MH, Norman AB, et al: Nicotine potentiation of haloperidol in reducing tic frequency in Tourette's disorder. Am J Psychiatry 148:793–794, 1991

McHenry LCJ: Samuel Johnson's tics and gesticulations. Journal of the History of Medicine 22:152–168, 1967

Meltzer HY, Matsubara S, Lee J-C: Classification of typical and atypical antipsychotic drugs on the basis of dopamine D-1, D-2 and serotonin pK values. J Pharmacol Exp Ther 251:238–246, 1989

Mikkelsen EJ, Detlor J, Cohen DJ: School avoidance and social phobia triggered by haloperidol in patients with Tourette's disorder. Am J Psychiatry 138:1572–1576, 1981

Murray TJ: Dr. Samuel Johnson's movement disorders. BMJ 1:1610–1614, 1979

Murray TJ: Doctor Samuel Johnson's abnormal movements, in Advances in Neurology, Vol 35, Gilles de la Tourette Syndrome. Edited by Friedhoff AJ, Chase TN. New York, Raven, 1982, pp 25–30

Nee LE, Caine ED, Polinsky RJ, et al: Gilles de la Tourette syndrome: clinical and family study in 50 cases. Ann Neurol 7:41–49, 1980

Nehra A: Pemoline-associated hepatic injury. Gastroenterology 99:1517–1519, 1990

Nomoto F, Machiyama Y: An epidemiological study of tics. Jpn J Psychiatry Neurol 44:649–655, 1990

Nomura Y, Segawa M: Gilles de la Tourette syndrome in Oriental children. Brain Dev 1:103–111, 1979

Nomura Y, Segawa M: Tourette syndrome in Oriental children: clinical and pathophysiological considerations, in Advances in Neurology, Vol 35, Gilles de la Tourette Syndrome. Edited by Friedhoff AJ, Chase TN. New York, Raven, 1982, pp 277–280

Nose T, Takemoto H: The effect of penfluridol and some psychotropic drugs on monoamine metabolism in central nervous system. Eur J Pharmacol 31:351–359, 1975

Nyback H, Schubert J, Sedvall G: Effect of apomorphine and pimozide on synthesis and turnover of labelled catecholamines in mouse brain. J Pharm Pharmacol 22:622–624, 1970

Opler LA, Feinberg SS: The role of pimozide in clinical psychiatry: a review. J Clin Psychiatry 52:221–233, 1991

Parikh MD, Abhyanka RR, Bajaj N, et al: Penfluridol in the treatment of Gilles de la Tourette's syndrome. Neurology (India) 27:174–177, 1979

Pasquier C, Pouplard F: Some thoughts on tics in children resulting from a therapeutic test. Revue de Neuropsychiatrie Infantile 25:645–651, 1977

Patel M: Letter to the editor: long-term neurologic complications of metaclopramide. N Y State J Med 3:210, 1986

Pauls DL, Towbin KE, Leckman JF, et al: Gilles de la Tourette's syndrome and obsessive-compulsive disorder: evidence supporting a genetic relationship. Arch Gen Psychiatry 43:1180–1182, 1986

Peroutka SJ, U'Prichard DC, Greenberg DA, et al: Neuroleptic drug interactions with norepinephrine alpha receptor binding sites in rat brain. Neuropharmacology 16:549–556, 1977

Pollera CF, Cognetti F, Nardi M, et al: Letter to the editor: sudden death after acute dystonic reaction to high-dose metoclopramide. Lancet 2:460–461, 1984

Price AR, Leckman JF, Pauls DL, et al: Tics and central nervous system stimulants in twins and non-twins with Tourette syndrome. Neurology 36:232–237, 1986

Regeur L, Pakkenberg B, Fog R, et al: Clinical features and long-term treatment of 65 patients with Gilles de la Tourette's syndrome. J Neurol Neurosurg Psychiatry 49:791–795, 1986

Ross MS, Moldofsky H: A comparison of pimozide and haloperidol in the treatment of Gilles de la Tourette's syndrome. Am J Psychiatry 1:103–111, 1978

Seeman P, Lee T: Antipsychotic drugs: direct correlations between clinical potency and presynaptic action on dopamine neurons. Science 188:1217–1219, 1975

Seignot MJN: Un cas de maladie des tics de Gilles de la Tourette gueri par le R-1625. Ann Med Psychol (Paris) 119:578–579, 1961

Shapiro AK, Shapiro E: Tics, Tourette Syndrome and Other Movement Disorders: A Pediatrician's Guide. New York, Tourette Syndrome Association, 1980

Shapiro AK, Shapiro E: Do stimulants provoke, cause or exacerbate tics and Tourette syndrome? Compr Psychiatry 22:265–273, 1981

Shapiro AK, Shapiro E: Controlled study of pimozide vs placebo in Tourette's syndrome. Journal of the American Academy of Child Psychiatry 23:161–173, 1984

Shapiro AK, Shapiro E: Evaluation of the reported association of obsessive-compulsive symptoms or disorder with Tourette's disorder. Compr Psychiatry 33:1–10, 1992

Shapiro AK, Shapiro E, Wayne HL: Treatment of Tourette's syndrome with haloperidol: review of 34 cases. Arch Gen Psychiatry 28:92–97, 1973

Shapiro AK, Shapiro E, Bruun RD, et al: Gilles de la Tourette Syndrome. New York, Raven, 1978

Shapiro AK, Shapiro E, Eisenkraft GJ: Treatment of Gilles de la Tourette syndrome with pimozide. Am J Psychiatry 140:1183–1186, 1983a

Shapiro AK, Shapiro E, Eisenkraft GJ: Treatment of Tourette disorder with penfluridol. Compr Psychiatry 24:327–331, 1983b

Shapiro AK, Shapiro E, Fulop G: Pimozide treatment of tic and Tourette disorders. Pediatrics 79:1032–1039, 1987

Shapiro AK, Shapiro E, Young JG, et al: Gilles de la Tourette Syndrome, 2nd Edition. New York, Raven, 1988

Shapiro E, Shapiro AK, Fulop G, et al: Controlled study of haloperidol, pimozide and placebo for the treatment of Gilles de la Tourette's syndrome. Arch Gen Psychiatry 46:722–730, 1989

Singer JS, Gammon K, Quaksey S: Haloperidol, fluphenazine and clonidine in Tourette syndrome: controversies in treatment. Pediatric Neurologic Science 12:71–74, 1986

Stevens H: Gilles de la Tourette and his syndrome by serendipity. Am J Psychiatry 128:489–492, 1971

Sverd J, Gadow KD, Paolicelli LM: Methylphenidate treatment of attention deficit hyperactivity disorder in a boy with Tourette syndrome. J Am Acad Child Adolesc Psychiatry 28:574–579, 1989

Sweet RD, Bruun RD, Shapiro E, et al: Presynaptic catecholamine antagonists as treatment for Tourette's syndrome. Arch Gen Psychiatry 31:857–861, 1974

Tibbits RW: Neuropsychiatric aspects of tics and spasms. Br J Hosp Med 25:454–457, 1981

Troung DD, Bressman S, Shale H, et al: Clonazepam, haloperidol, and clonidine in tic disorders. South Med J 8:1103–1105, 1988

Trousseau A: Des diverses especes de chorees. Clinique Medicale de l'Hotel Dieu (Paris) 2:264–271, 1873

Uhr SB, Berger PA, Pruitt B, et al: Treatment of Tourette's syndrome with R022-1319, a D-2 receptor antagonist (letter). N Engl J Med 311:989, 1984

Uhr SB, Pruitt B, Berger PA, et al: Case report of four patients with TS treated with piquindone, a D2 receptor antagonist. J Clin Psychopharmacol 6:128–130, 1986

Van Woert MH, Rosenbaum D, Enna SJ: Overview of pharmacological approaches to therapy for Tourette syndrome, in Advances in Neurology, Vol 35, Gilles de la Tourette Syndrome. Edited by Friedhoff AJ, Chase TN. New York, Raven, 1982, pp 369–375

Wassman ER, Eldridge R, Abuzzahab FS Sr, et al: Gilles de la Tourette syndrome: clinical and genetic studies in a midwestern city. Neurology (Minneap) 28:304–307, 1978

Yusuf S, Wittes J, Probstfield J, et al: Analysis and interpretation of treatment effects in subgroups of patients in randomized clinical trials. JAMA 266:93–96, 1991

CHAPTER 8

Cognitive Effects of Neuroleptic Use in Children With Tourette's Syndrome

Floyd R. Sallee, M.D.
Christina M. Rock, B.S.
Lori A. Head, Pharm.D.

In this chapter, we address differences in the way that two of the major neuroleptic medications used in the treatment of Tourette's syndrome (TS), haloperidol and pimozide, may affect cognitive performance and school functioning. When these medications were first introduced for the treatment of the involuntary motor and vocal tics associated with the disorder, it became apparent that extrapyramidal side effects would limit their utility. The doses initially recommended corresponded to chlorpromazine equivalents (CPZ-EQ) of 1,000–2,000 mg/day. These doses were based largely on the literature associated with the use of haloperidol and pimozide in the schizophrenic population, and the assumption was made that the occupancy of the same dopaminergic receptors was involved. This led to a widespread perception of cognitive dulling and clinical depression associated with the use of these medications. Clinical dosage titration to eliminate tics was limited by a definite ceiling effect attributed to severe extrapyramidal side effects.

When clinicians applied these adult dosage regimens to children, reports of anxiety disorders, school phobic symptoms, and frank depression (Bruun 1988) became apparent either as dosage was being titrated upward or after several months on a stable maintenance dose. This would indicate that the therapeutic index or the range of dose between therapeutic and toxic thresholds is rather narrow in children. Cognitive blunting is often associated with neuroleptic use in TS (Erenberg 1988), but formal neuropsychological batteries are apparently insensitive to medication effects (Bornstein and Yang 1991). Despite these potential problems, neuroleptics do improve certain aspects of mental functioning if used in lower doses (Werry and Aman 1975). These authors were the first to describe the potential benefits of low-dose haloperidol treatment in improving errors of commission on a Continuous Performance Test (CPT) and improving search efficiency in a memory searching task in children. Although data concerning laboratory task performance has been obtained, the relationship between laboratory task performance and school performance for children exposed to neuroleptics has been limited.

Haloperidol (Haldol), the current treatment of choice in TS, was approved for use in children with TS in 1978. It is efficacious in 90% of cases, with tic symptom reduction in the range of 60%–80% (Bruun 1984; A. K. Shapiro et al. 1973, 1983). The dosage must be titrated against an endpoint of incapacitating side effects compared with relief of tics. Haloperidol produces side effects in the motor (extrapyramidal), cognitive (attention, memory, learning), and affective (lethargy, phobia, depression) domains in a high percentage of patients. In 50% of patients treated with haloperidol, significant side effects either interfere with therapeutic effects or nullify them to the degree that patients must be removed from the medication (Erenberg 1988; A. K. Shapiro et al. 1973). Reports by Bruun (1988) and others would indicate that haloperidol-associated dysphoria itself may result in poor school performance. Interfering side effects may appear at relatively low doses of haloperidol of 1–6.5 mg/day. Haloperidol treatment may impair motivation, decrease attention, and impair learning, but careful studies showing such problems are few (Goldstone and Lhamon 1976; Goldstone et al. 1979; Platt et al. 1981, 1984). In a more recent study by E. Shapiro et al. (1989), 20% of the patients treated with a mean daily dose of haloperidol of 4.5 ± 2.7 mg (100–350 mg CPZ-EQ) reported moderate or marked loss of motivation, depression, and/or cognitive dulling.

Pimozide, the first "orphan" drug approved under the 1983 Orphan Drug Amendments to the Federal Food, Drug, and Cosmetic Act, has been claimed as an alternative to haloperidol in the treatment of TS. Although pimozide is more than four times as potent as haloperidol in the treatment of schizophrenia and five times more potent at binding to the D_2 receptor (Pinder et al. 1976; Seeman 1980), its relative potency in TS has yet to be established. Studies suggest that pimozide has an efficacy comparable to (and perhaps greater than) haloperidol for relief of TS and is associated with fewer adverse neuropsychiatric and extrapyramidal side effects (Ross and Moldofsky 1978; A. K. Shapiro and Shapiro 1984; E. Shapiro and Shapiro 1982). In our experience, pimozide produces many of the same adverse reactions as haloperidol, but at a much higher dosage level, with a wider therapeutic index. Pimozide also produces a characteristic activation of the central nervous system as reported in the adult literature (Pinder et al. 1976). Pimozide has many advantages over haloperidol that may recommend it as the drug of first choice in the treatment of this disorder. One reservation about the use of pimozide in TS, particularly with children, concerns cardiac side effects. An electrocardiographic abnormality associated with pimozide use involves the rate-corrected QT interval (QTc or the time during which the heart contracts and relaxes). Prolongation of the QTc interval increases the risk of potentially fatal arrhythmia. A study by Fulop et al. (1987) demonstrated that although the QTc increased with pimozide treatment, the increase was not clinically significant, and no adverse effects were noted in 40 patients with TS.

Differences in the therapeutic and toxic consequences of haloperidol and pimozide treatment may be due to differences in their mechanism of action. Haloperidol seems to affect both pre- and postsynaptic receptor sites, whereas pimozide seems to act at postsynaptic sites only (Borison et al. 1981; Walters and Roth 1975). It has been shown that chronic administration of neuroleptics such as haloperidol, which block presynaptic dopamine receptors (Walters and Roth 1975), induces alterations in dopamine synthesis and release that may contribute to the development of conditions such as tardive dyskinesia. When postsynaptic receptors become supersensitive (Sayers et al. 1975) with chronic neuroleptic drug use, continued treatment with a presynaptic blocker such as haloperidol may be disadvantageous in that more transmitter is produced to compete at the supersensitive postsynaptic site, leading to toxicity. Unlike haloperidol, pimozide acts preferentially at the postsynaptic dopamine receptor. Overutilization of pimozide and haloperidol may increase the risk of tardive dyskinesia (E. Shapiro and Shapiro 1982). Although it has been thought that many withdrawal dyskinesias induced by these treatments are limited in patients with TS, a report by Riddle et al. (1987) indicated that tardive dyskinesia is a genuine risk in TS patients.

Pimozide, a diphenylbutylpiperidine, is also a potent calcium-channel blocker, which could account for its activating effects (Gould et al. 1983). An explanation of the toxic effects of both drugs on behavior and cognitive functioning may be that the plasma concentrations are extremely high despite the oral dose given. We have reported several adult patients treated with pimozide who have had toxic reactions after several months of treatment on low-dose pimozide because of extremely long biological half-lives (Sallee et al. 1987). The present literature does not examine a possible relationship between plasma drug concentration and toxic consequences on behavior and cognition. Indeed, there is no generally accepted therapeutic plasma level range for haloperidol in TS, and no information exists at present on pimozide. Morselli et al. (1979) suggested a therapeutic range for haloperidol in TS of 1–6 ng/ml, whereas Singer et al. (1982), using a nonspecific radioreceptor assay, reported a therapeutic range of 1–4 ng/ml. If therapeutic and toxic plasma level ranges were established for haloperidol and pimozide, variability of patient response and overutilization of these drugs could be controlled.

The following open assessment of haloperidol versus pimozide was conducted in a sample of 63 children with a confirmed diagnosis of DSM-III-R (American Psychiatric Association 1987) Tourette's disorder. In the open trial, children were evaluated in a tertiary care TS specialty outpatient clinic often after multiple neurological evaluations. A subset were under medication treatment at the time of the evaluation. The strategy of the study was to compare the treatment groups within 3 weeks of presentation to the clinic in terms of school performance and behavior as well as laboratory cognitive measures of vigilance and memory search efficiency. The main inferences to be evaluated were whether neuroleptic treatment at clinically relevant therapeutic doses had a positive or adverse effect on cognitive performance.

Methods

Sixty-three children with a confirmed diagnosis of DSM-III-R Tourette's disorder were consecutively referred from an outpatient clinic and evaluated by a child psychiatrist using the Tourette Symptom Global Scale (Harcherik et al. 1984). The most common comorbid diagnosis (44%) was attention-deficit/hyperactivity disorder (ADHD). The overwhelming majority were males (n = 57, 90.5%), with an age range of 7–15 years (mean age, 10.5 ± 2.5). These patients were referred by their pediatrician, psychiatrist, or neurologist to a tertiary care clinic specializing in the care of TS. While on medication of at least 6 months' duration, 38 patients presented to the clinic; 16 were on haloperidol, and 22 were on pimozide. Of the subset of medication-treated patients, 38% had comorbid ADHD but were treated with neuroleptic alone. The mean treatment doses of haloperidol and pimozide were 1.5 ± 0.6 mg/day (45–105 CPZ-EQ) and 3.7 ± 1.4 mg/day (76–168 CPZ-EQ), respectively. Teacher reports of school functioning and behavior were elicited for 44 of the children through the use of the Child Behavior Checklist—Teacher Report Form (CBCL-TRF) (Achenbach and Edelbrock 1983) within 3 weeks of evaluation. At the second clinic visit, all children completed a cognitive test battery consisting of a CPT adapted to the Apple IIe microcomputer (Lindgren and Lyons 1984) and 47 children also received a memory search task (Sternberg 1969).

Continuous Performance Test

The CPT, developed by Lindgren and Lyons (1984), was used in a colorless presentation. A series of capital letters are shown on the screen for a time period varying from 100 to 120 milliseconds. (Variation in time is caused by fluctuation in the monitor scanning.) When an *H* appeared on the screen immediately followed by a *T*, the subject was required to press the space bar before the next two letters appeared. No response was required for any other letter combination. Omission and commission errors per session are reported for the CPT. Duration of the task was 15 minutes.

Memory Search Task

In the memory search task, subjects were asked to memorize a set of letters containing either one, three, or six stimuli, which are scattered in the squares of a 3×3 grid. These stimuli constitute the positive set, which is referred to as the memory load. Memory load was the independent variable, with the dependent variable being the reaction time. Both reaction time and error rate as well as linear reaction time memory load function are calculated. Slope and intercept of a linear reaction time load function are the data reported for the memory search task. Length of the task was 20 minutes.

Data Analysis

Group data (no drug, haloperidol, pimozide) with respect to CPT errors (omission and commission) were compared by analysis of variance (ANOVA). Due to variability in teacher compliance, only 54 responses were obtained, of which 44 were considered valid; the CBCL-TRF was considered invalid if six of the items went unanswered. The 19 patients who were not included in the CBCL-TRF analysis did not differ in age, IQ, TS severity, presence of comorbid ADHD, or CPT errors from the subset of 44. School behavior and academic performance data from the CBCL-TRF were analyzed by ANOVA as T-scores. Internalizing and externalizing dimensions were compared across medicated and nonmedicated groups. Subscales for all behavioral dimensions and for academic functioning were analyzed across medicated and nonmedicated groups by ANOVA, with particular emphasis on the following items: VII (academic performance relative to grade level); selected items from VIII, including "how hard is he/she working" and "how much is he/she learning" relative to others in the classroom; and a sum of all items from VIII, including a component of classroom behavior.

Results

Mean dose of neuroleptic adjusted for body weight was 1.5 mg (75 mg CPZ-EQ) or 0.05 mg/kg/day for haloperidol and 4.2 mg (138.6 mg CPZ-EQ) or 0.14 mg/kg/day for pimozide. In the haloperidol group, this dose achieved a total haloperidol plasma level of 2.6 ± 1.4 ng/ml, which was well within the acceptable therapeutic range reported (Morselli et al. 1979; Singer et al. 1982). The no-drug group (n = 25) did not significantly differ from the pimozide (n = 22) or haloperidol (n = 16) groups with respect to age or tic symptom severity (mean Tourette Symptom Global Scale score, 27). Mean ages in years for the groups were 10.8 (no drug), 10.4 (haloperidol), and 10.8 (pimozide). Those patients who were treated with pimozide did differ with respect to their performance on the CPT (see Table 8–1). Errors of commission were lower in the pimozide-treated group (1.5 ± 3.1) compared with the haloperidol-treated group (5.3 ± 7.1) and no-drug group (4 ± 4.6) (P < .05). Errors of omission did not differ across groups.

A subset of patients from each group (haloperidol = 10, pimozide = 17, no drug = 20) received the memory search task. Drug-treatment groups tended toward increased efficiency of memory search (lower intercept value), but group differences were not statistically significant based on ANOVA. No differences in slope were demonstrated across groups. Figure 8–1 illustrates the group data, which are plotted as mean reaction time across the three memory loads (one, three, six stimuli).

School performance data based on teacher ratings on the CBCL-TRF from a subset of 44 of the 63 children are presented in Table 8–2. Although this was a subsample, it was determined that

Table 8–1. Continuous Performance Test errors

Group	*n*	Omissions	Commissions
No drug	25	5.5 ± 6.8	4.0 ± 4.6
Haloperidol	16	5.3 ± 6.9	5.3 ± 7.1
Pimozide	22	4.0 ± 4.6	1.5 ± 3.1[a]

[a]Significantly different from no-drug group (P < .05) and from haloperidol group (P < .05).

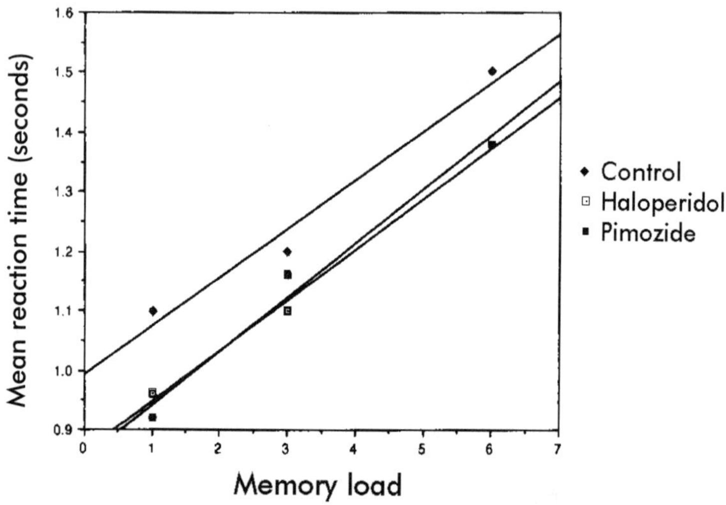

Figure 8–1. Memory processing efficiency is illustrated from the memory search task as group means plotted for each treatment group. The linear reaction time (RT) memory load function is similar for the neuroleptics haloperidol and pimozide, with enhanced performance in memory search efficiency (intercept) over no-drug control group; slope of the RT function is unchanged.

Table 8–2. Teacher-rated school performance mean adaptive functioning T-score

		Child Behavior Checklist—Teacher Report Form item			
Group	***n***	**VII School performance**	**VIII-1 Working hard**	**VIII-3 Learning**	**VIII-4 Total function**
No drug	19	43	51	49	46
Haloperidol	12	44	41[a]	42[b]	39[b]
Pimozide	13	46	49[c]	48	45

[a]Significantly different from no-drug group ($P < .005$).
[b]Significantly different from no-drug group ($P < .05$).
[c]Significantly different from haloperidol group ($P < .05$).

no systematic bias excluded the remainder of the group and that this subset accurately reflected the entire sample in terms of age, IQ, TS severity, ADHD comorbidity, and CPT performance. Differences between drug-treatment groups were detected in teacher ratings of perceived academic performance. Haloperidol-treated children were perceived by their teachers as giving inferior effort, with less learning capacity and poorer academic functioning than either the pimozide-treated or the no-drug groups. Haloperidol-treated children (n = 12/16) differed from the pimozide-treated children (n = 13/22) in the category "working hard" (ANOVA, $P < .05$). The haloperidol-treated children also differed from the no-drug group (n = 19/25) in the categories "working hard" (ANOVA, $P < .05$), "learning" (ANOVA, $P < .05$), and total academic function (ANOVA, $P < .05$). Groups did not differ in age, IQ, tic symptom severity, or comorbidity of ADHD. Drug treatment did not seem to impact on school behavior, with no group differences on either externalizing or internalizing dimensions and their respective subcategories.

Discussion

The fact that many TS children have comorbid ADHD (44% in this sample) is often used as a justification for the use of clonidine as an alternative to neuroleptics (Leckman et al. 1991). We have found that certain aspects of cognitive functioning, such as memory search efficiency and CPT errors, do improve with low-dose neuroleptics. Pimozide seems effective in improving not only laboratory measures of functioning but can be viewed as not interfering with performance in the classroom. Performance of children on low-dose haloperidol was less than optimal, with teacher reports showing decreased academic functioning in the classroom in categories of "working hard," "learning," and "total function," compared with the no-drug condition. Medicated patients differed in the category "working hard," with pimozide showing significantly higher teacher ratings of performance compared with haloperidol. Classroom behaviors in both the internalizing and externalizing dimensions remained unchanged by drug treatment. Differences in school performance between groups were not due to effects of haloperidol or pimozide on mood or on motivation. Bruun (1988) suggested the dysphoric effect of haloperidol is the result of the external anxiety caused by an unfamiliar situation overriding the internal distress caused by the situation. As school is a more novel environment than home, negative effects of haloperidol might be more prominent in this environment. There is some support for this from animal studies. Sanberg and Norman (1989) discovered that rats in a habituated environment that are injected with haloperidol had an increased emotional response and those in a novel environment had a typical "dysphoric" response. These findings would argue for a complex interaction between haloperidol and the environment, with the outcome dependent on the emotional state of the individual.

Selective attention appears to be mediated through the dopaminergic system (Cheal 1984). D_2 blocking agents like haloperidol and pimozide in low doses have been shown to enhance latent learning in animals (Ichihara et al. 1989). This effect is best attributed to action at the D_2 postsynaptic receptor because selective blockade of the D_2 autoreceptor alone, as with sulpiride, disrupts passive avoidance learning (Ichihara et al. 1988), and D_1 blocking suppresses learning and inhibits exploratory behavior. Therefore, the positive effects on elements of learning demonstrated in our studies with children with TS might come from action at the D_2 receptor, although other pharmacological sites of action are certainly involved. Differences between pimozide and haloperidol might stem from unique pharmacological profiles of the two drugs. Pimozide is pharmacologically distinct from haloperidol in that it possesses the capacity to down regulate D_2 receptors after chronic treatment, whereas haloperidol up regulates D_2 receptor number (Tecott et al. 1986). Furthermore, pimozide possesses significant calcium-channel blocking ability (Gould et al. 1983) and exhibits little of the alpha-adrenergic blocking activity attributed to haloperidol. Pimozide belongs to the verapamil-like class of calcium antagonists and selectively modulates L-type calcium channels (King et al. 1989). This may explain in part its distinct action to attenuate both the positive and negative symptoms of schizophrenia and why pimozide is frequently activating in patients, whereas haloperidol is frequently sedating.

A previous study by Bornstein and Yang (1991) that compared the neuropsychological performance of medicated and unmedicated TS children found no difference between those children taking psychotropic medication and the no-drug group. The medicated group, however, was predominantly clonidine treated, and few patients were receiving neuroleptics. In the present open study, we have avoided inclusion of clonidine-treated children because of their milder TS symptoms. Because Bornstein and Yang did not use a measure of tic severity, it cannot be determined conclusively if subjects in our study compare with those of Bornstein and Yang. Of their medicated subjects, 48% were taking clonidine, but no differentiation is made in their data between subjects on haloperidol, pimozide, and clonidine. Although both studies used low-dose medicated subjects, findings from neuropsychological laboratory testing showed little or no difference between medicated and unmedicated groups. The present study went a step further, including school teacher perceptions of performance, which showed marked differences, especially for the haloperidol group. The negative attributes of some neuroleptic treatments, especially haloperidol, may be elicited only from observers witnessing these children functioning in complex environments (e.g., classroom), which cannot be duplicated by laboratory tasks such as the CPT. A teacher's perception of less learning taking place and less effort being expended by the haloperidol-treated children may be a reflection of subtle cognitive effects or sedation occurring in conjunction with treatment. More work needs to be done to determine in what situations the cognitive dulling caused by haloperidol is most detrimental.

References

Achenbach TM, Edelbrock CS: Manual for the Child Behavior Checklist and Revised Child Behavior Profile. Burlington, University of Vermont Department of Psychiatry, 1983

American Psychiatric Association: Diagnostic and Statistical Manual of Mental Disorders, 3rd Edition, Revised. Washington, DC, American Psychiatric Association, 1987

Borison RL, Fields JZ, Diamond BI: Site specific blockade of dopamine receptors by neuroleptic agents in human brain. Neuropharmacology 20:1321–1322, 1981

Bornstein RA, Yang V: Neuropsychological performance in medicated and unmedicated patients with Tourette's Disorder. Am J Psychiatry 148:468–471, 1991

Bruun RD: Gilles de la Tourette's syndrome: an overview of clinical experience. Journal of the American Academy of Child Psychiatry 23:126–133, 1984

Bruun RD: Subtle and under recognized side effects of neuroleptic treatment in children with Tourette's disorder. Am J Psychiatry 145:621–624, 1988

Cheal ML: Differential effects of haloperidol and clozapine on attention. Psychopharmacology 84:268–273, 1984

Erenberg G: Pharmacologic therapy of tics in childhood. Pediatr Ann 17:395–404, 1988

Fulop G, Phillips RA, Shapiro AK, et al: ECG changes during haloperidol and pimozide treatment of Tourette's disorder. Am J Psychiatry 144:673–675, 1987

Goldstone S, Lhamon WT: The effects of haloperidol upon temporal information processing by patients with Tourette's Syndrome. Psychopharmacology (Berlin) 50:7–10, 1976

Goldstone S, Nurnberg HG, Lhamon WT: Effects of trifluoperazine, chlorpromazine, and haloperidol upon temporal information processing by schizophrenic patients. Psychopharmacology (Berlin) 65:119–124, 1979

Gould RJ, Murphy KM, Reynolds IJ, et al: Antischizophrenic drugs of the diphenylbutylpiperidine type act as calcium channel antagonists. Proc Natl Acad Sci U S A 80:5122–5125, 1983

Harcherik DF, Leckman JF, Detlor J, et al: A new instrument for clinical studies of Tourette's syndrome. Journal of the American Academy of Child Psychiatry 23:153–160, 1984

Ichihara K, Nabeshima T, Kameyama T: Effects of haloperidol, sulpiride, and SCH 23390 on passive avoidance learning in mice. Eur J Pharmacol 151:435–442, 1988

Ichihara K, Nabeshima T, Kameyama T: Differential effects of pimozide and SCH 23390 on acquisition of learning in mice. Eur J Pharmacol 164:189–195, 1989

King VF, Garcia ML, Shevell JL, et al: Substituted diphenylbutylpiperidines bind to a unique high affinity site on the L-type calcium channel: evidence for a fourth site in the cardiac calcium entry blocker receptor complex. J Biol Chem 264:5633–5641, 1989

Leckman JF, Hardin MT, Riddle MA, et al: Clonidine treatment of Gilles de la Tourette's syndrome. Arch Gen Psychiatry 48:324–328, 1991

Lindgren SD, Lyons DA: Pediatric Assessment of Cognitive Efficiency (PACE). Iowa City, University of Iowa, Department of Pediatrics, 1984

Morselli PL, Bianchetti G, Durand G, et al: Haloperidol plasma level monitoring in pediatric patients. Ther Drug Monit 1:35–46, 1979

Pinder RM, Brogan RN, Sawyer PR: Pimozide: a review 26 of its pharmacological properties and therapeutic uses in psychiatry. Drugs 12:1–40, 1976

Platt JE, Campbell M, Green WH, et al: Effects of lithium carbonate and haloperidol on cognition in aggressive hospitalized school-age children. J Clin Psychopharmacol 1:8–13, 1981

Platt JE, Campbell M, Green WH, et al: Cognitive effects of lithium carbonate and haloperidol in treatment resistant aggressive children. Arch Gen Psychiatry 41:657–662, 1984

Riddle MA, Hardin TM, Towbin KE, et al: Tardive dyskinesia following haloperidol treatment in Tourette's syndrome. Arch Gen Psychiatry 44:98–99, 1987

Ross MS, Moldofsky H: A comparison of pimozide and haloperidol in the treatment of Gilles de la Tourette's syndrome. Am J Psychiatry 135:585–587, 1978

Sallee FR, Pollock BG, Stiller RL, et al: Pharmacokinetics of pimozide in adults and children with Tourette's syndrome. J Clin Pharmacol 27:776–781, 1987

Sanberg PS, Norman AB: Underrecognized and underresearched side effects of neuroleptics. Am J Psychiatry 146:411–412, 1989

Sayers AC, Burki HR, Ruch W, et al: Neuroleptic-induced hypersensitivity of striatal dopamine receptors in the rat as a model of tardive dyskinesias: effects of clozapine, haloperidol, loxapine, and chlorpromazine. Psychopharmacology (Berlin) 41:97–104, 1975

Seeman S: Brain dopamine receptors. Pharmacol Rev 32:229–313, 1980

Shapiro AK, Shapiro E: Controlled study of pimozide vs placebo in Tourette's syndrome. Journal of the American Academy of Child Psychiatry 23:161–173, 1984

Shapiro AK, Shapiro E, Wayne H: Treatment of Tourette's syndrome with haloperidol: review of 34 cases. Arch Gen Psychiatry 28:92–97, 1973

Shapiro AK, Shapiro EE, Eisenkraft MA: Treatment of Gilles de la Tourette syndrome with pimozide. Am J Psychiatry 140:1183–1186, 1983

Shapiro E, Shapiro AK: Tardive dyskinesia and chronic neuroleptic treatment of Tourette patients. Adv Neurol 35:413–414, 1982

Shapiro E, Shapiro AK, Fulop G, et al: Controlled study of haloperidol, pimozide, and placebo for the treatment of Gilles de la Tourette's syndrome. Arch Gen Psychiatry 46:722–730, 1989

Singer HS, Butler IJ, Tune LE, et al: Dopaminergic dysfunction in Tourette syndrome. Ann Neurol 12:361–366, 1982

Sternberg S: Memory scanning: mental process revealed by reaction time experiments. Am Sci 57:421–457, 1969

Tecott LH, Kwong LL, Uhr S, et al: Differential modulation of dopamine D_2 receptors by chronic haloperidol, nitrendipine and pimozide. Biol Psychiatry 21:1114–1122, 1986

Walters JR, Roth RH: Dopaminergic neurons: alterations in the sensitivity of tyrosine hydroxylase to inhibition by endogenous dopamine after cessation of impulse flow. J Pharmacol Exp Ther 25:649–654, 1975

Werry J, Aman MG: Methylphenidate and haloperidol in children: effects on attention, memory, and activity. Arch Gen Psychiatry 32:790–795, 1975

CHAPTER 9

Neuroleptic-Induced Behavior Disorders in Patients With Tourette's Syndrome

Ruth Dowling Bruun, M.D.
Cathy L. Budman, M.D.

Prior to the 1960s, Tourette's syndrome (TS) was conceptualized as an essentially psychological disorder. Because its etiology was attributed to various psychodynamic conflicts and nonspecific constitutional factors, treatment strategies emphasized psychotherapy and other nonpharmacological approaches. Treatment outcomes were often dismally disappointing, and many TS patients remained debilitated by their symptoms throughout life, ostracized to a great extent by the community. It was only after the discovery that haloperidol could effectively treat certain symptoms of TS that a neuropsychiatric basis for this disorder became more widely accepted (Shapiro et al. 1973). The availability of a more specific treatment for TS heralded a surge of renewed scientific interest and investigation into this intriguing illness.

Because treatment with haloperidol led to clinical improvement in the majority of TS patients (Bruun 1984; Shapiro et al. 1983), there was initially considerable enthusiasm for its use. Because little was known about both neuroleptics and the complexities of symptoms in TS in the 1970s, early pharmacological goals focused almost exclusively on eliminating as many tics as possible. Although these early drug trials in TS patients often employed considerably higher neuroleptic doses than in subsequent years, an interesting phenomenon soon emerged: Most patients preferred having tics to experiencing the side effects of neuroleptic treatment. Furthermore, many TS patients seemed to have symptoms of behavioral and motor toxicity even on low doses of haloperidol.

One of the more distressing side effects described by many patients treated with neuroleptics is a sense of mental dulling. The possibility of neuroleptic-induced cognitive blunting was investigated in TS patients in the late 1970s and early 1980s with conflicting results (Bogomolny et al. 1982; Goldstone and Lhamon 1976). However, as more TS patients were treated with haloperidol, evidence began to accumulate that this agent was associated with impaired attention, motivation, and memory (Shapiro and Shapiro 1988). In the mid-1980s, the antipsychotic pimozide, which is chemically similar to haloperidol, was demonstrated to cause slowing of performance and memory impairment in TS patients when compared with placebo (Shapiro et al. 1988).

As more time passed, a variety of side effects were reported in TS patients treated with neuroleptics, including lethargy, weight gain, extrapyramidal symptoms, dysphoria, depression, outbursts of aggression and violence, work avoidance, and phobic behavior (Bruun 1982; Linet 1985; Mikkelsen et al. 1981). It remains unclear whether some of these problems actually represent epiphenomenon of neuroleptic-induced akathisia because decompensation, violence, and suicidal ideation have been attributed to akathisia in at least some patients treated with neuroleptics (Keckich 1978; Shaw et al. 1986; Van Putten et al. 1974).

Interestingly, among patients who are treated with neuroleptics for psychiatric disorders, there appears to be a subpopulation of patients who are either unchanged or who actually become worse with conventional neuroleptic therapy. Neuroleptic-related psychotic exacerbations were first reported by Simpson et al. in 1976; they felt that these symptoms either reflected "an exacerbation of the condition for which the neuroleptic was being administered or may be a side effect of the neuroleptic" (p. 367). Although the literature describes several cases of neuroleptic-induced psychotic exacerbation in psychotic patients treated with haloperidol (Bowers and Swigar 1988; Tornatore et al. 1981), the prevalence of this problem is not known at the present time.

Although these clinical observations suggest the possibility of neuroleptic side effects manifesting as behavioral disturbances, this has received little systematic evaluation. In our experience, neuroleptic side effects may be manifested by behaviors such as outbursts of hostility, poor socialization, promiscuity, antisocial acts, withdrawal, and suicidal ideation, and it is often difficult to distinguish such behavioral side effects from underlying psychopathology. Unfortunately, this is further complicated by the fact that many TS patients have associated behavioral symptoms that themselves appear, evolve, and remit over time (Comings and Comings 1987; Singer and Rosenberg 1989). Thus, careful assessment of individual cases must be done to exclude the possibility of concomitant psychopathology as the primary cause of such symptoms.

Over the past 20 years, one of us (R.B.) has had the opportunity to treat many children with TS who were not psychotic or acutely disturbed prior to being given neuroleptics. Such cases facilitate identification of subtle neuroleptic side effects presenting as behavioral problems (Bruun 1988). The possibility of spontaneous onset of associated psychopathology cannot be ruled out in all cases. However, recurrence of symptoms after rechallenge with neuroleptics in certain cases supports the hypothesis that these symptoms are neuroleptic related.

In our clinical experience, we have treated 33 children, ranging in age from 7 to 20 years, with symptoms meeting DSM-III-R (American Psychiatric Association 1987) criteria for the diagnosis of TS, who have been treated with neuroleptics (usually haloperidol or pimozide) and who presented behavioral problems that remitted with either discontinuation or reduction of the neuroleptic dosage. These behavioral problems were insidious in nature, gradually evolving into patterns consistent with diagnoses of oppositional defiant disorder, conduct disorder, depression, or an anxiety disorder. Of these patients, 21 received haloperidol, 9 received pimozide, 1 received fluphenazine, and 2 received sequential treatment with pimozide and haloperidol or with pimozide and fluphenazine at the time they developed behavioral disturbances. The sex distribution in this cohort was 6 girls and 27 boys, which approximates the distribution by sex of TS in the general population (Robertson 1989). The majority of the children ($n = 22$) were over age 12, which may reflect the greater reluctance to employ neuroleptic medication in younger patients with TS. In contrast to the more commonly recognized extrapyramidal side effects, behavioral symptoms developed slowly and increased in severity with time on medication. Concurrent use of anticholinergic medications did not alleviate these behavioral symptoms. The children themselves were often not aware of any adverse effects of medication while they were manifesting the behavioral symptoms; only in retrospect were they able to describe their difficulties.

Illustrative Cases

The following cases illustrate what we believe to be symptoms of behavioral toxicity associated with neuroleptic treatment.

Case 1

Rick began having tics at age 4 while being treated with methylphenidate for attention-deficit/hyperactivity disorder. By age 8 the tics were severe, and a diagnosis of TS was made. Methylphenidate was discontinued, and haloperidol was given instead. During the next few years, it became apparent that although low doses of haloperidol were fairly effective, higher doses caused a worsening of TS symptoms such as coprolalia and copropraxia.

Until the age of 16, Rick was maintained on 2.5 mg/day of haloperidol or less. Although he disliked the sedation, he felt a need for medication to control his tics. When pimozide became available, he was eager to try it. Initially, he felt better on this medication and denied any side effects. Soon afterward, Rick began to have more trouble getting along with his family; he was described as uncooperative, immature, and defiant at home. He also started having school problems. His marks began to drop, and he had difficulty socializing with his peers. He became involved in disruptive, even dangerous, activities such as setting fires and playing silly pranks. His psychologist felt that he had a "fragile ego" and could not cope with his illness. As time passed, he became increasingly immature, lacking in motivation and unable to handle any responsibility. A child psychiatrist who was consulted gave the opinion that he had a "severe personality disorder."

Rick entered college but was asked to leave after only 2 months because of antisocial behavior, which included lying, stealing, gambling, urinating, and masturbating in an exhibitionistic fashion. After leaving college, he obtained several jobs but was unable to keep them because he refused to follow orders and stole small sums of money. Later the same year, he entered a residential program for "children who have lost control of their lives." While he was there (for almost 2 years), pimozide was gradually increased to a maximum of 8.5 mg/day. He was unable to progress at all in the program. His own attempt to participate consisted of admitting to drug abuse, a fabrication he concocted to "fit in better."

After leaving the residential program, Rick returned home. He expressed his hopelessness and anger in writing: "hatred is what I am . . . ready to explode . . . come death . . . you could be the family that died to me years ago." Shortly after this time, he stopped taking pimozide. Within 2 weeks, he felt like "a different person." Within a couple of months, he was working full-time in the family business and taking classes at night. He gradually regained self-esteem and learned to socialize in a more mature manner. His tics also diminished.

The contrast between Rick when medicated with pimozide and when unmedicated only a few months later was striking. When he was asked to describe the subjective changes on medication versus off medication, he said that while on pimozide he had ceased to care what happened to him. He could not sustain attention and had almost no frustration tolerance. He lacked empathy for other people and had little interest in forming relationships. Rather, he felt irritable most of the time and simply wanted to be left alone. He estimated that 80%–90% of those negative feelings disappeared when the medication was stopped. The remaining changes he attributed to increased self-esteem and maturity. Although normal maturation may have contributed to Rick's personality change, it seemed, in retrospect, that the neuroleptic paralyzed him in a regressed state that could have been perceived superficially as psychodynamically determined. This state may have been produced by neuroleptic-induced akinesia, dysphoria, cognitive or affective blunting, or other subtle side effects.

Case 2

James first developed tics at age 5, and TS was diagnosed at age 11 when tics became marked. Over the next 5 years, he was treated with haloperidol in doses up to 16 mg/day, but his tics were only partially controlled. James became listless, had trouble concentrating in school, lost all motivation for academics, and complained of insomnia at night and daytime drowsiness. He was always tired in the mornings and often missed school or was late. As his academic performance deteriorated, he became increasingly depressed. He attempted suicide at age 12 by throwing himself out of a car. At age 14, he attempted suicide three more times by overdoses and was hospitalized for several weeks. Haloperidol dosage was gradually reduced at this time, and antidepressants (imipramine and subsequently doxepin) were prescribed.

At age 16, haloperidol was discontinued, and James was treated with pimozide. (Trials on clonazepam and clonidine had been unsuccessful.) At a dose of 12 mg/day of pimozide, James began to have explosive temper outbursts during which he broke furniture, threatened family members, and hurt himself by punching walls and putting his fist through windows. He also had several episodes of intense anxiety during which he suddenly went into a dissociative state, assuming the identity of his grandfather in a concentration camp in 1944. At that time, it was suggested that pimozide might be responsible for the behavioral disturbances. However, the patient told his parents that he had been abusing mescaline and requested admission to a psychiatric hospital.

Once in the hospital, James admitted that he had fabricated the story of substance abuse in a desperate attempt to obtain help. The doctors at the hospital viewed him as behaving "hysterically." They saw "no connection between his behavior and the pimozide except for his emotional reaction to being medicated." Psychological testing revealed "confusion around identity conflicts" and "a struggle to fulfill [his] distorted perceptions of a male role." Pimozide was raised to 20 mg/day, and carbamazepine, clonazepam, and benztropine were added. He was discharged without any significant change in his emotional state.

When James returned home, he was even more explosive. He seemed to get more anxious and restless toward the end of each day; his outbursts usually occurred in the evenings. His mother was fearful of being alone with him, but both parents were extremely reluctant to lower the pimozide dosage. They felt that if he was partially out of control on this dosage, he would be completely out of control on less medication. However, because his tics were now quite mild, they finally consented to an attempt to taper the pimozide slowly.

Pimozide was reduced over the next 4 months to 8.0 mg/day. At this dose, James was "perhaps better." His mother was not certain whether he was less explosive or if he was simply spending more time out of the house with friends. However, over the next several months, the family life began to return to normal. James had no more dissociative states. Then he experienced a waxing of tics, and coprolalia became prominent. James increased his pimozide dosage at his own initiative back to 12 mg/day, but he became explosive once again. He withdrew socially, paced constantly at home, and threatened to burn the house down. It was not clear what had caused this decompensation until James admitted he had increased his medication. When he was persuaded to decrease the dose to 10 mg/day, his symptoms abated, predictably, about 5 days later.

James has since had periodic tic exacerbation and has tried at least twice more to raise pimozide above 10 mg/day. On each occasion, he began to feel more angry and frightened. Hence, he has discontinued all other medications and remains on lower doses of pimozide.

James' experiences with neuroleptics were different from Rick's, mainly in that James expressed his internal dysphoria with more overt affect. Although Rick's feelings of hopelessness and apathy were acted out mostly through passive antisocial behaviors, James' despair was more dramatically demonstrated by suicidal gestures and aggression. Nonetheless, there were striking similarities between the two cases. Both boys chose to invent stories of substance abuse because they felt that such problems would be better understood by their parents and their doctors than the more ambiguous feelings they were actually experiencing. It is ironic that they chose to blame illicit drugs for their behaviors when it appears that they were actually experiencing side effects of prescribed medications.

Case 3

Sara had tics beginning at age 4, and at age 8 TS was diagnosed. She was treated with clonidine, which initially seemed effective. However, a few months later, Sara developed loud coprolalia, and haloperidol was substituted for clonidine. Coprolalia was controlled, but Sara gained weight very rapidly. In an effort to avoid obesity, haloperidol was replaced by pimozide 4 months later. While coprolalia continued to be controlled, Sara now began to exhibit copropraxia, which upset her, her teachers, and her family. Despite medical advice to the contrary, Sara's mother increased the dose of pimozide to 20 mg/day. Sara's copropraxia did not improve, and coprolalia returned.

Sara became a discipline problem in school and refused to cooperate with class activities. Soon, her hostile and destructive behavior manifested itself at home too. She teased and physically abused her dog, fought with her siblings, and finally had a rage attack during which she cut up most of her clothes. When she was brought to the physician's office, she had almost constant, loud coprolalia and many simple and complex motor tics. She was extremely irritable, which contrasted markedly with her previously pleasant affect.

When it was discovered that Sara had been taking such a high dose of pimozide, the dose was immediately decreased by half. A week later, Sara's mother reported an improvement both in her TS symptoms and behavior. For the next 3 years, Sara did quite well on a combination of pimozide (10 mg/day) and clonazepam (0.5 mg bid). Although coprolalia persisted, it was relatively mild. Sara's greatest concern was her weight, which continued to be excessive. However, she was popular with schoolmates and seemed happy at home.

At age 13, TS symptoms again became quite severe. Once more, Sara's mother began giving Sara increased doses of pimozide. Two months later, Sara began to complain that she was under too much pressure at school, although her teachers reported that the work load had not changed. Sara was tired all the time and often went to bed after dinner. She became more clingy, irritable, and miserable. Her grades dropped precipitously. Two months later, Sara reported she had heard voices telling her to hit herself in her head. Her mother became frightened and agreed to discontinue pimozide, which was lowered rapidly and then discontinued. After pimozide was stopped, Sara became "a different child altogether." Her TS symptoms have been severe at times but nonetheless she has been coping extremely well. She lost the excess weight, has showed renewed interest in schoolwork, and is popular with her peers. She has not experienced subsequent hallucinatory experiences.

As with the case of James, rechallenge with increased doses of a neuroleptic caused a recurrence of behaviorally manifested drug side effects: outburst of rage punctuated by periods of despair, apathy, and fear. The hallucinatory experience she described was unusual; it is not clear whether this was an episode of transient psychosis, a sensory tic, obsessive-compulsive thinking, or a regressive response to severe dysphoria. By her own account, Sara felt confused and frightened by her behavior at the time.

Case 4

Jennifer developed symptoms of TS when she was 3, and the diagnosis of TS was made when she was 8. During the next 6 years, her symptoms waxed and waned in typical fashion but were never troublesome enough to require treatment with medication.

However, during the summer when she was 15, both motor and vocal tics became severe. A trial of clonidine was unsuccessful. Just before school started in the fall, she was placed on treatment with fluphenazine up to 3 mg/day. There was considerable improvement initially but then her tics worsened. Fluphenazine was raised to a level of 5 mg/day. The immediately apparent side effects included an acute dystonic reaction (which responded to benztropine) and an 18-pound weight gain.

Her family observed that Jennifer was more emotionally labile and difficult to get along with and attributed this to the increase in her TS symptoms and a recent breakup with a boyfriend. Although Jennifer had previously been a good student, she now found it difficult to do her homework and to attend school. She often came home after only one or two classes. Soon she began to stay home for several days at a time because she "felt too sick" (from severe tics, muscle aches, fatigue, and nausea).

Her medication was changed from fluphenazine to pimozide

6 mg/day. However, she became even more "moody." She began to experience severe sleep disturbances (was unable to fall asleep until 5 A.M.) and consequently was too fatigued to attend school. She had tantrums at home and crying spells while in school. Pimozide was changed to haloperidol 4 mg/day. Attempts to taper the dose were unsuccessful because the tics increased with decreasing dosages. Her teachers and her family felt that she was not trying to cope with school but Jennifer insisted that no one understood how hard she was truly pushing herself.

Although she had once enjoyed reading, Jennifer now found it an "excruciating experience." Writing one-page book reports took days of effort. At the same time, Jennifer also began to behave quite promiscuously, although this was ego-dystonic and left her feeling "cheap and immoral." By the spring term, Jennifer could not attend school at all. Sometimes she got as far as the front hall at school only to turn around and go home. She deliberately isolated herself from her former friends and began identifying herself with "losers"—the only people with whom she now felt comfortable. Her tics continued to be severe. In desperation Jennifer further increased haloperidol to 8 mg/day and on occasions took even higher doses. At home she began to have physical fights with her parents and on occasion pleaded with them to take her to a hospital. She told her doctor that she felt there was nothing to live for. A home tutor was arranged but Jennifer still refused to do any schoolwork.

Then, in June, Jennifer became ill with a gastrointestinal virus and was unable to take any medication for over a week. During this period she began to feel "strangely well . . . almost like my old self." However, after she recovered, she resumed taking haloperidol and soon lapsed back into "the miasma." She spent hours writing gloomy poetry but could not do any work for her final exams. Three weeks later she was finally persuaded to decrease her medication. By mid-July she was down to 2 mg/day of haloperidol, and her tics remained unchanged. She surprised herself and her parents by getting a summer job in a music store. By mid-August she stopped haloperidol completely. She began to take more pride in her appearance and by fall returned to school with renewed enthusiasm and motivation.

Since then, Jennifer has done well academically and has returned to her previous social milieu. She describes herself when on medication as feeling "like a cactus, dry and prickly inside and outside." Now, off medication, she feels "more like a rose. There are still a few thorns but it's beautiful anyway." Her tics are severe at times but she copes well with them.

This case, too, illustrates the loss of motivation, the low frustration tolerance, and the pervasive dysphoria that seem to generate antisocial acting-out behaviors. Like the patients in the other cases, Jennifer demonstrated a striking change in personality that appeared directly related to neuroleptic medication.

Discussion

In this chapter, we described four cases that exemplify what appear to be behavioral problems secondary to side effects of neuroleptic therapy. We have observed such a relationship in 33 children with TS who were treated with neuroleptic medications, primarily haloperidol or pimozide. Behavioral disturbances included lying, stealing, explosive outbursts of hostility, hurting or threatening to hurt others, promiscuity, poor socialization, immature or regressive behaviors, and suicidal ideation. Although haloperidol was employed in the majority of cases at the time behavior problems developed, this most likely reflects the overall greater use of this agent in the TS population. All of these patients improved markedly when neuroleptic treatment was discontinued or the neuroleptic dose was lowered. Treatment with anticholinergic medication did not appear to relieve the behavioral symptoms.

Although one could argue that neuroleptics induce or unmask underlying behavioral problems, we believe these behaviors are in themselves consequences of neuroleptic side effects. Certainly extrapyramidal symptoms and akathisia are common, often disturbing, side effects of these medications (Donlon and Stenson 1976). It appears that younger patients may be more vulnerable to parkinsonian side effects of moderate doses of haloperidol (Moleman et al. 1986), and such side effects might contribute to the behavioral disturbances we observed. However, one would expect that anticholinergic medication would ameliorate such symptoms, and this was clearly not the case. It is more difficult to rule out the possibility that these behavioral symptoms were related to akathisia, which has been documented to be associated with both suicide attempts and violence (Drake and Ehrlich 1985; Keckich 1978).

It is also difficult to dismiss fully the possibility of concurrent psychopathology. However, if underlying psychopathology existed, one would expect such character traits to endure with time, and this was not the case. Instead, what we observed was the insidious appearance of behavioral disturbances while these patients were treated with neuroleptics and the resolution of these behavior problems with the cessation or lowering of neuroleptic dosage.

There has been much recent interest in behavioral disturbances that are thought to be associated with TS. Such associated symptoms include obsessive-compulsive disorder, attention-deficit/hyperactivity disorder, aggressiveness, withdrawal, depression, conduct disorder, oppositional behaviors, panic attacks, phobias, and learning difficulties (Comings and Comings 1985, 1987; Robertson et al. 1988; Singer and Rosenberg 1989; Singer and Walkup 1991). Although some or all of these problems may be inherent to TS, we would suggest that the same or similar behaviors may be caused by treatment with neuroleptic medication. Certain features of apparent psychotic exacerbation with neuroleptics, such as depressed mood, guilt, and fears of death or of imminent tragedy (Bowers and Swigar 1988), seen in psychotic populations seem to occur also in some patients with TS who are treated with these agents. In addition, a variety of insidious antisocial behaviors may occur, as we have described. Because neuroleptic medication is so frequently used to treat symptoms of TS as well as a variety of unrelated psychiatric conditions, the possibility that these drugs can play a primary role in inducing and exacerbating the very behaviors for which they are often prescribed warrants further investigation.

References

American Psychiatric Association: Diagnostic and Statistical Manual of Mental Disorders, 3rd Edition, Revised. Washington, DC, American Psychiatric Association, 1987

Bogomolny A, Erenberg A, Rothner AD: Behavioral effects of haloperidol in young Tourette syndrome patients, in Advances in Neurology, Vol 35: Gilles de la Tourette Syndrome. Edited by Friedhoff AJ, Chase TN. New York, Raven, 1982, pp 427–432

Bowers MB Jr, Swigar ME: Psychotic patients who became worse on neuroleptics. J Clin Psychopharmacol 8:417–421, 1988

Bruun RD: Dysphoric phenomena associated with haloperidol treatment of Tourette syndrome, in Advances in Neurology, Vol 35: Gilles de la Tourette Syndrome. Edited by Friedhoff AJ, Chase TN. New York, Raven, 1982, pp 433–436

Bruun RD: Gilles de la Tourette syndrome: an overview of clinical experience. Journal of the American Academy of Child Psychiatry 23:126–133, 1984

Bruun RD: Subtle and underrecognized side effects of neuroleptic treatment in children with Tourette's disorder. Am J Psychiatry 145:621–624, 1988

Comings DE, Comings BG: Tourette syndrome: clinical and psychological aspects of 250 cases. Am J Hum Genet 37:435–450, 1985

Comings DE, Comings BG: A controlled study of Tourette syndrome I-VII. Am J Human Gen 41:701–866, 1987

Donlon PT, Stenson RL: Neuroleptic induced extrapyramidal symptoms. Diseases of the Nervous System 37:629–635, 1976

Drake RE, Ehrlich J: Suicide attempts associated with akathisia. Am J Psychiatry 142:499–501, 1985

Goldstone S, Lhamon WT: The effects of haloperidol upon temporal information processing by patients with Tourette's syndrome. Psychopharmacology (Berlin) 50:7–10, 1976

Keckich WA: Neuroleptics: violence as a manifestation of akathisia. JAMA 240:2185, 1978

Linet LS: Tourette syndrome, pimozide and school phobia: the neuroleptic separation anxiety syndrome. Am J Psychiatry 142:613–615, 1985

Mikkelsen EJ, Detlor J, Cohen DJ: School avoidance and social phobia triggered by haloperidol in patients with Tourette's disorder. Am J Psychiatry 138:1572–1576, 1981

Moleman P, Janzen G, von Bargen B, et al: Relationship between age and incidence of parkinsonism in psychiatric patients treated with haloperidol. Am J Psychiatry 143:232–234, 1986

Robertson M: The Gilles de la Tourette syndrome: the current status. Br J Psychiatry 154:147–169, 1989

Robertson M, Trimble MR, Lees AJ: The psychopathology of the Gilles de la Tourette syndrome: a phenomenological analysis. Br J Psychiatry 152:383–390, 1988

Shapiro AK, Shapiro E: Treatment of tic disorders with haloperidol, in Tourette's Syndrome and Tic Disorders. Edited by Cohen DJ, Bruun RD, Leckman JF. New York, Wiley, 1988, pp 268–280

Shapiro AK, Shapiro E, Wayne H: Treatment of Tourette's syndrome with haloperidol: review of 34 cases. Arch Gen Psychiatry 28:92–97, 1973

Shapiro AK, Shapiro E, Eisenkraft GJ: Treatment of Gilles de la Tourette syndrome with clonidine and neuroleptics. Arch Gen Psychiatry 40:1235–1240, 1983

Shapiro AK, Shapiro E, Young JG, et al: Gilles de la Tourette Syndrome. New York, Raven, 1988

Shaw ED, Mann JJ, Weiden PJ, et al: A case of suicidal and homicidal ideation and akathisia in a double-blind neuroleptic crossover study. J Clin Psychopharmacol 6:196–197, 1986

Simpson GM, Varga E, Haher J: Psychotic exacerbations produced by neuroleptics. Diseases of the Nervous System 37:367–369, 1976

Singer HS, Rosenberg LA: The development of behavioral and emotional problems in Tourette syndrome. Pediatr Neurol 5:41–44, 1989

Singer HS, Walkup JT: Tourette syndrome and other tic disorders: diagnosis, pathophysiology and treatment. Medicine 70:15–32, 1991

Tornatore FL, Lee D, Sramek JJ: Psychotic exacerbation with haloperidol. Drug Intelligence and Clinical Pharmacy 15:209–218, 1981

Van Putten T, Mutalipassi LR, Malkin MD: Phenothiazine-induced decompensation. Arch Gen Psychiatry 30:102–105, 1974

APPENDIX

Cross-Referenced List of Selected Medications Used in This Book

Generic name	Brand name(s)	Indication
Amantadine	Symmetrel	Antiparkinson
Amoxapine	Asendin	Antidepressant
Benztropine	Cogentin	Antiparkinson
Chlorpromazine	Thorazine	Antipsychotic
Chlorprothixene	Taractan	Antipsychotic
Clozapine	Clozaril	Antipsychotic
Diazepam	Valium	Antianxiety
Diphenhydramine	Benadryl	Antiparkinson
Fluphenazine	Prolixin	Antipsychotic
Haloperidol	Haldol	Antipsychotic
Loxapine	Loxitane	Antipsychotic
Mesoridazine	Serentil	Antipsychotic
Methylphenidate	Ritalin	Antihyperactivity
Molindone	Moban	Antipsychotic
Perphenazine	Trilafon, Etrafon	Antipsychotic
Pimozide	Orap	Antipsychotic (tics)
Prochlorperazine	Compazine	Antipsychotic
Thioridazine	Mellaril	Antipsychotic
Thiothixene	Navane	Antipsychotic
Trifluoperazine	Stelazine	Antipsychotic

Index

Page numbers printed in **boldface** *type refer to tables or figures.*

Abbreviated Dyskinesia Rating Scale (ADRS), 122, 129
Abnormal Involuntary Movement Scale (AIMS), 3, 76, 122, 129
Abnormal involuntary movements, 36, 99, 186
  assessment for, 46
  in children with autism, 121–133
    haloperidol for, 128–132
    neuroleptic-related dyskinesias, 125–128
    stereotypies, 121–125
  criterion symptoms for, **44**
  demographic and behavioral characteristics of subjects evaluated for, 49–50, **50–51**
  expected responses to changes in medication status, **49**
  individual case atypicality of, 44–45, 51, **52–54, 59,** 59–63
    causes of, 59
  methods for study of, 45–49
  prevalence of, 44–45
  related to neuroleptic chlorpromazine-equivalent dose and anticholinergic activity, **52–54,** 55–59
  tic disorders, 137–164
Academic impairment, 86, 87, 162, 172, 192
Acetophenazine, **47**
ADHD (attention-deficit/hyperactivity disorder), 2–3, **8,** 32, **50,** 58, 85
Adjustment disorder, **50,** 57
  gender and neuroleptic dosage for, 29, 31, **31**
  gender distribution of, 28
  prevalence of psychotropic drug use for
    gender differences in, 29, **30**
    related to length of hospitalization, 25
ADRS (Abbreviated Dyskinesia Rating Scale), 122, 129
Affective blunting, 72, **79,** 162, 189
Affective disorders
  gender and neuroleptic dosage for, 29, 31, **31**
  gender distribution of, 28
  prevalence of psychotropic drug use for
    gender differences in, 29, **30**
    related to length of hospitalization, 25
Age effects, 28, 35
Aggressiveness, 2, 5, **7,** 12, 85, 186, 195, 196
Agranulocytosis, 154–155

AIMS (Abnormal Involuntary Movement Scale), 3, 76, 122, 129
Akathisia, 143, 145, 186, 195–196
Akinesia, 143, 145, 162, 189
Alcohol abuse, 45, **50**
Allergic desensitization, 147
Alpha-methylparatyrosine, for tic disorders, 145
Amantadine, 58, 199
American Hospital Formulary Service, 27
Aminobutyric acid inhibitors, 147
Amitriptyline, **48,** 146
Amotivation, 172, 186, 188, 195
Amoxapine, 55, 199
  anticholinergic activity factor for, **48**
  chlorpromazine-equivalent dose of, **47**
Analysis of variance (ANOVA), 28, 32, 35, 176, 179
Anorexia, 16
Anticholinergic activity factors, **48,** 48–49
Anticholinergic drugs, xxi, 195
  effect on tardive dyskinesia, 62
  gender differences in use of, 29, **30,** 38
  prevalence of use among hospitalized patients, 24–25
Anticonvulsants, 146
  gender differences in use of, **30**
Antidepressants, 146, 162
  gender differences in use of, 29, **30**
Antisocial behavior, 189
Anxiety, 187
  gender distribution of, 28
  phobias, 161–162, 172, 186, 196
  separation anxiety disorder, 114, 161
Anxiolytics, 146
  gender differences in use of, **30**
Apomorphine, 146
Arson, 45, **51,** 62
Artane. *See* Trihexyphenidyl
Asendin. *See* Amoxapine
Assaultiveness, 45, 50, **51**
Assessment of patients. *See also* Monitoring of patients
  baseline, xxiv, 3
  instruments for, 1–2
  during neuroleptic treatment for tic disorders, 154–156
  during study of haloperidol for schizophrenia, 76
Attention
  decreased, 172, 186
  selective, 180
  sustained, 90–91
Attention-deficit/hyperactivity disorder (ADHD), 2–3, **8,** 32, **50,** 58, 85
  haloperidol for, 3, **8**
  neuropsychological testing in, 159
  stimulants for, 32, 139
    in patients with comorbid Tourette's disorder, 156–159
  thioridazine for, 3, 32
  Tourette's disorder and, 156–158, 175, 179, 196
Autism, xx, 2
  differentiation of infantile autism from schizophrenia, 70–71
  haloperidol for, **9,** 74, 123–126, **124,** 128–132
    design of study of, 128–129
    findings from long-term study of, 129–130

neuroleptic-related dyskinesias in children with, 125–128
overview of neuroleptics for, 5, **6**, **7**, **9–11**, 12
pimozide for, 3, **11**, 12
selecting neuroleptics for, xxii
stereotypies in children with, 121–125. *See also* Stereotypies

Baclofen, 147
Baseline assessments, xxiv, 3
Behavioral problems, 2, **6**, 86
Tourette's disorder and, 159–160, 196
Behavioral toxicity of neuroleptics, xxiii, 2, 14, 34–36, 185–196
case studies of, 188–195
Benadryl. *See* Diphenhydramine
Benefits of neuroleptics, xx
Benzodiazepines, 146, 147
Benztropine, 55–58, 146, 190, 199
anticholinergic activity factor for, **48**
Beta-blockers, 146
Bipolar disorder, 5, 72
Bleuler, E., 67
Blood dyscrasias, 143
Botulinum serum injections, 148
Brief Psychiatric Rating Scale for Children (BPRS-C), 76, 78
Butaperazine, **47**

Calcium-channel blockers, 147, 174, 180
Carbamazepine, 27, 146, 190
Child Behavior Checklist—Teacher Report Form (CBCL-TRF), 175, 177, **178**
Children's Psychiatric Rating Scale (CPRS), 2, 76, 78, 99–101, 107–108, **108–109**, 122, 129
Chlordiazepoxide, 146
Chlorimipramine, 146
Chlorpromazine, 1, 28, 58, 199
for aggressiveness, 85
anticholinergic activity factor for, **48**
for attention-deficit/hyperactivity disorder, 3
for conduct disorder, aggressive type, 12–13
for delusional depression, 5, **7**
effect on seizure threshold, 3, 126
for hyperactivity and aggressiveness, **7**
for schizophrenia, 71–72
for tic disorders, 143
Chlorpromazine equivalents, **47**, **52–54**
Chlorprothixene, 28, **47**, 199
Choline, 146
Cholinergic agonists, 146
Cholinergic antagonists, 146
Clinical Global Impressions (CGI), 76, 78, **78–79**, 103, 105, 150
Clinical trials, lack of, 23–24
Clonazepam, 147, 190, 192
Clonidine, for Tourette's disorder, 147, 181, 192
comorbid with attention-deficit/hyperactivity disorder, 158, 179
Clorazepate, 146
Clozapine, 199
anticholinergic activity factor for, **48**
dosage of, 70

Clozapine *(continued)*
for schizophrenia, 5, **11,** 70, 73
side effects of, 145
for tic disorders, 145
Clozaril. *See* Clozapine
Cogentin. *See* Benztropine
Cognitive effects of neuroleptics, xxii–xxiii, 12
in children with conduct disorder, 85–114
in children with mental retardation, 13
in children with Tourette's disorder, 161, 171–181, 186
measurement of, 87–98
Continuous Performance Test, 89–98, 175–179
related to dosage, 88, 98, 171–172
study of haloperidol and pimozide, 171–181
Continuous Performance Test, 175–179, **177–178**
design, 174–175
dosage, 175, 177
mechanisms of action, 173–174
subject selection, 175
study of molindone and thioridazine, 98–111
behavior changes, 107–109, **108–110**
behavior ratings, 103, 105–106
clinical implications of, 113–114
Continuous Performance Test procedures, 103–104
Continuous Performance Test results, 109–112, **110**
design, **102,** 102–103
dosage, 103, 106
limitations of, 112–113
results, 105–111
side effects, 106–107
statistical analyses, 105
subject selection, 99–101, **101**
Cogwheel rigidity, 78
Compazine. *See* Prochlorperazine
Compliance. *See* Noncompliance
Computer applications, xxiv, 87
Conduct disorder, 2, **50,** 58, 187, 196
aggressive type, 12–13
cognitive effects of neuroleptics used for, 85–114. *See also* Cognitive effects of neuroleptics
diagnosis of schizophrenia in patients hospitalized for, 32
gender and neuroleptic dosage for, 29, 31, **31,** 32
gender distribution of, 28
haloperidol for, **8, 12–13,** 74
overview of neuroleptics for, **8, 10,** 12–13
prevalence of psychotropic drug use for
gender differences in, 29, **30,** 32–33
related to length of hospitalization, 25
rationale for neuroleptic use in, 32–33
Conners Abbreviated Parent-Teacher Questionnaire, 103, 107, **108–109,** 149–150
Conners Parent-Teacher Questionnaire, 2, 76

Conners Teacher Questionnaire, 76, 100
Continuous Performance Test (CPT), xxiii, xxiv, 89–98, 172, 175–179
  analysis of data from, 92, **93,** 176
  ceiling effects on, 109, 111
  clinical applications of, 89
  construct validity of, 90
  dynamic, 92–96, **95**
  errors of omission and commission on, 91, **91,** 92, 94, **95**
  face validity of, 89
  interstimulus interval (ISI) for, 90, 94–96, **95**
  measurement of sustained attention by, 90–91
  medication effects on, 98
    sensitivity to amphetamine drug effects, 89–90
    sensitivity to neuroleptic drug effects, 112
  playing card version of, 91–92
  response demands of, 91
  signal detection and, 96–98
  to study effects of haloperidol and pimozide, 175–179
    memory search task, 176, **178**
    procedures, 175–176
    results, **177–178,** 177–179
  to study effects of thioridazine and molindone
    procedures for, 103–105
    results of, 109–112, **110**
  test-retest reliability of, 90
Coprolalia, 86, 188, 192
Copropraxia, 188, 192
Corticosteroids, 147
Crying spells, 161, 194
Crystalluria, 145

Deanol, 146
Decompensation, 186, 191
Delusions, 72, 74, 77, **79**
Dementia praecox, 67–68
Depersonalization, 162
Depot neuroleptics, 15
Depression, **50,** 55, 61, 161, 162, 172, 186, 187, 196
  atypical, **50**
  delusional, 5, **7**
Dermatitis, 143
Desipramine, **48,** 146, 158
Dextroamphetamine, 2, 87, 159
Diagnosis
  criteria for, 2, 35
  related to age and gender, 28–29, 33, 35
Diagnostic Interview for Children and Adolescents—Revised, 76
Diaphoresis, 16
Diarrhea, 16
Diazepam, 146, 199
Diet, 147
Diltiazem, 147
Diphenhydramine, **48,** 58, 78, 199
Disruptive behavior, 2, **6**
Disulfiram, for tic disorders, 146
Dizziness, 78, 107
Dopamine agonists, 146
Dopamine antagonists
  D_2 blocking agents, 180
  for tic disorders, 144–146
Dosage, xxi, xxii. *See also* specific drugs
  atypical tardive dyskinesia and parkinsonism related to, **52–54,** 55–59, 63
  chlorpromazine equivalency, **47**

Dosage *(continued)*
cognitive effects related to, 88, 98, 171–172
compliance and, 15
gender differences in, 25–26, 29, 31, **31,** 33
implications of increasing over time, 34
lack of research information on, 23–24
maximum, 3
overmedication, 14
psychological cap on, 43
related to length of hospitalization, 24–25
schedule for, 3, **4**
starting, 3
for treating tic disorders, 151–152
Dosage Order Treatment Emergent Symptoms Scale (DOTES), 103
Doxepin, **48,** 190
Drooling, 78
Drowsiness, 78, 145, 192
Drug abuse, 45, **50**
fabricated history of, 189–191
Drug tolerance, 34
Dyskinesias, neuroleptic-associated, 12, 16, 143. *See also* Tardive dyskinesia
in children with autism, 125–128
initial, 62
repeated, 130–132
treatment-emergent, 63, 131–132
withdrawal, 3, 12, 63, 127, **127,** 174
repeated, 130–132
risk factors for, 130
Dysphoria, 161, 162, 172, 180, 186, 189, 191–195
Dystonia, 78, 99, 107, 114

Elavil. *See* Amitriptyline
Electrocardiogram (ECG), 76
monitoring during desipramine treatment, 158
monitoring during pimozide treatment, 155–156
Electroconvulsive therapy, 147
Electroencephalogram (EEG), 76
Enuresis, 145
Estrogens, 36–37
Ethosuximide, 146
Etrafon. *See* Perphenazine
Explosiveness, 2, 12, 190–191, 195
Eye blinking, 122, 148

Fantasies, 162
Fatigue, 194
Fenfluramine, for stereotypies, 125
Finger movements, 122
Fluoxetine, 146
Fluphenazine, 28, **47,** 56, 58, 199
anticholinergic activity factor for, **48**
for autism, **6, 7**
chlorpromazine-equivalent dose of, **47**
for schizophrenia, 72
for tic disorders, xxiii, 142–143, 152–154, 187, 193
Flurazepam, 146
Fog states, 86, 147, 162–163
Frustration intolerance, 189

Gambling, 189
Gastric upset, 107

Gender differences, 23–28
  methods for study of, 26–28
  in neuroleptic dosage, 25–26, 29, 31, **31**
  in neuroleptic use among hospitalized patients, 29, **30**
  in prevalence of atypical parkinsonism, 60–61
  in prevalence of neuroleptic-related dyskinesias, 130
  in prevalence of tardive dyskinesia, 36
  related to age and diagnosis, 28, 35
  results of study of, 28–31
  univariate analyses of, 28–29
  in use of high- versus low-potency neuroleptics, 33–34, 38
Global Clinical Judgments consensus ratings, 77, 78
Grimacing, 122

Haldol. *See* Haloperidol
Hallucinations, 72, 74, 77, **79**, 192–193
Haloperidol, 28, 56, 58, 199
  for aggressiveness, 85
  anticholinergic activity factor for, **48**
  for attention-deficit/hyperactivity disorder, 3, **8**
  for autism, **9**, 74, 123–126, **124**, 128–132
  for conduct disorder, **8**, 12–13, 74
  dosage of, 3, **4**, 69, 76, 77, 79, 123, **124**, 130, 172
    chlorpromazine-equivalent dose, **47**
    therapeutic range for, 174
  indications for, 4
  mechanism of action of, 173–174
  for schizophrenia, 5, **7**, **8**, 67–80
    assessing response to, 76–77
    design of study of, 75–77
    effectiveness of, 77–80, **78–79**
    reasons for selection of, 74
    subject selection for study of, 74–75
  side effects of, 78, 172–173
    behavioral toxicity, 185–196
    cognitive effects, 88, 98, 171–181
    dyskinesias, 12
    in school versus at home, 180, 181
  for stereotypies, 123–125, **124**
  for tic disorders, xxii, xxiii, **9**, 140–141, 152–154, 172
Hand flapping, 122
Head banging, 122
Headache, 107
Hepatitis, 154
Holistic treatment, 147
Homicidal ideation, 74
Hospitalization, psychiatric
  family history of, 46, 50, **51**
  gender differences in neuroleptic use during, 23–38, **30**
  haloperidol for schizophrenia during, 73–80
  prevalence of psychotropic drug use related to length of, 24–25
L-5-Hydroxytryptophan, 146
Hyperactivity, 2, 5, **6**, **7**, 45, **51**, 85–86, 99

Imipramine, **48,** 146, 158, 190
Impulsivity, 99
Indications for neuroleptics, xix–xxi, 2–3, 86, 114
  unlabeled, 36
Information processing, 87. *See also* Cognitive effects of neuroleptics
Informed consent, 75, 159
Inpatient Aggression Scale (IAS), 100, 103, 107, **108–109**
Insulin coma therapy, 147
Intelligence quotient (IQ) of autistic children
  haloperidol effects on, 12
  relation of stereotypies to, 122–123
Irritability, 2, 12, 99, 161, 192

Jaundice, 154
Judgment impairment, 74

Kolvin, I., 70–71
Kraepelin, E., 68

Language therapy, 12
Learning. *See* Cognitive effects of neuroleptics
Learning disorders, 196
Lecithin, 146
Lethargy, 145, 162, 172, 186
Leukopenia, 145
Levodopa, 146
Lip movements, 122
Literature review of neuroleptic use in children, **6–11,** 23–24
  for schizophrenia, 69–73
Lithium, 146
  for aggressiveness, 12, 85
  for conduct disorder, 12
  gender differences in use of, 29, **30**
Liver dyscrasias, 143
Loxapine, 199
  anticholinergic activity factor for, **48**
  chlorpromazine-equivalent dose of, **47**
  dosage of, 69
  for schizophrenia, 69
Loxitane. *See* Loxapine
Ludiomil. *See* Maprotiline
Lying, 189, 195

"Maladie des tics," 138
Malpractice claims, 159
Maprotiline, **48**
Masklike facies, 78
Masturbation, 189
Matching Familiar Figures Task, 87
Megavitamins, 147
Mellaril. *See* Thioridazine
Memory impairment, 87, 186
Mental retardation, 2, **6, 11,** 13, 122
Mesoridazine, 28, 199
  anticholinergic activity factor for, **48**
  chlorpromazine-equivalent dose of, **47**
Methylphenidate, 2, 32, 73, 158, 188, 199
  effect on cognitive tasks, 87, 88
Metoclopramide, 145
  for tic disorders, 144
Moban. *See* Molindone
Molindone, 28, 56, 57, 99, 199
  anticholinergic activity factor for, **48**
  for autism, **10**
  chlorpromazine-equivalent dose of, **47**
  cognitive effects of, 98–111. *See also* Cognitive effects
  for conduct disorder, **10,** 13
  dosage of, 99, 106

effectiveness of, 99
for schizophrenia, 73
side effects of, 99
Monitoring of patients, xxiv, 14–15, 154–156
Monoamine oxidase, 60–61
Monoamine oxidase inhibitors, 146

Naltrexone
for stereotypies, 125
for tic disorders, 147
Naturalistic studies, 24
Nausea, 16
Navane. *See* Thiothixene
Neuroleptic malignant syndrome, 86
Neuroleptics
behavioral toxicity, xxiii, 2, 14, 34–36, 185–196
case studies of, 188–195
cognitive effects of, 85–114
compliance with, 15–16
depot, 15
gender differences in use of, 23–38, **30**
high-potency versus low-potency, 3, 28, 33–34, 125–126
gender differences in use of, 33–34, 38
prolactin response induced by, 38
indications for, xix–xxi, 2–3, 86, 114
literature review of use in children, **6–11,** 23–24, 69–73
monitoring patient on, xxiv, 14–15, 154–156
prescribing practices for, 24
prevalence of use related to length of hospitalization, 24–25
taking history of use of, 46
Nifedipine, 147
Noncompliance, 46, 107
detection of, 16
due to side effects, 15, 37–38, 43
reasons for, 15
Norpramin. *See* Desipramine
Nortriptyline, **48**
Nurse's Global Impressions, 76

Observation of patients, 14–15. *See also* Monitoring of patients
Obsessive-compulsive symptoms or disorder (OCS-OCD), 139
tic disorders and, 159–160, 196
Oppositional defiant disorder, 187
Orap. *See* Pimozide
Orphan Drug Act, 141, 173
Orthomolecular mineral therapy, 147
Outpatient treatment issues, 14–16, 24
compliance, 15–16
monitoring, 14–15
Overmedication, 14

Paired Associates Task, 87, 88
Pamelor. *See* Nortriptyline
Panic attacks, 196
Paranoid states, 162, 163
Parkinsonism, xxiii, 36, 44, 143, 195
affective symptomatology and vulnerability to, 60, 62
criterion symptoms for, **44**
evaluation for, 46

Parkinsonism *(continued)*
expected responses to changes in medication status, **49**
individual case atypicality of, 44–45, 51, **52–54, 59,** 59–63
gender differences in, 59–61
methods for study of, 45–49
monoamine oxidase and, 60–61
noncompliance related to, 38
prevalence of, 45
related to neuroleptic chlorpromazine-equivalent dose and anticholinergic activity, **52–54,** 55–59
Penfluridol, for tic disorders, 142, 154
Periorbital movements, 122
Perphenazine, 28, 143, 199
anticholinergic activity factor for, **48**
chlorpromazine-equivalent dose of, **47**
Personality disorders
gender and neuroleptic dosage for, 29, 31, **31**
prevalence of psychotropic drug use for
gender differences in, 29, **30**
related to length of hospitalization, 25
Pharmacodynamics, 24
Pharmacokinetics, 24
Phenothiazines, **6–7.** *See also* specific drugs
side effects of, 143
for tic disorders, 142–144
Phenytoin, 146
Phobias, 161–162, 172, 186, 196
Photosensitivity, 143
Physical abuse, 45–46, **51**
Physostigmine, 146
Pimozide, 28, 199
for autism, 3, **11,** 12
behavioral toxicity of, 185–196
cautions about use of, 155
cognitive effects of, 171–181
electrocardiogram monitoring during treatment with, 155–156
mechanism of action of, 174
for mental retardation with disruptive behavior, **11**
pharmacology of, 180
potency compared with haloperidol, 173
for schizophrenia, 3, 69
for tic disorders, xxii, xxiii, **11,** 12, 141–142, 152–154, 173
Piperacetazine, **47**
Piperazines, **6–7**
Piperidines, **6**
Piquindone, for tic disorders, 146
Porteus Maze, 87, 88, 98
Prescribing practices, 24
Pribedil, 146
Primidone, 146
Prochlorperazine, 143, 199
anticholinergic activity factor for, **48**
chlorpromazine-equivalent dose of, **47**
Prolactin response, 38
Prolixin. *See* Fluphenazine
Promiscuity, 194, 195
Propranolol, 27
Psychological therapy, 148
Psychoses, 2. *See also* Schizophrenia
exacerbated by neuroleptics, 186–187
infantile versus late-onset childhood, 70–71

Psychosocial functioning, 162
Psychotropic drugs
American Hospital Formulary Service classification of, 27
utilization among hospitalized patients, 29, **30**

Quide. *See* Piperacetazine

Rage attacks, 192
Recall, 87
Regressive behavior, 195
Repoise. *See* Butaperazine
Research information, lack of, 23–24, 68–69
Reserpine, 145
Residential placement, 189
Restlessness, 99
Rigidity, cogwheel, 78
Ritalin. *See* Methylphenidate
Rocking, 122
Running away, 45, **51**

Sadness, 161
Salivation, 145
Schizoaffective disorder, **50**, 72–73
Schizophrenia, xx, xxi, 2, 5, **50**, 57, 68
age at onset of, 72
clozapine for, 5, **11**, 70, 73
diagnosis of, 68
differentiation from infantile autism, 70–71
efficacy of neuroleptics for, 23
gender and neuroleptic dosage for, 29, 31, **31**, 36–37
haloperidol for, 5, **7**, **8**, 67–80
assessing response to, 76–77
design of study of, 75–77
dosage of, 76, 77, 79
effectiveness of, 77–80, **78–79**
reasons for selection of, 74
side effects of, 78
subject selection for study of, 74–75
historical recognition in children, 67–68
importance of longitudinal follow-up of, 73
literature review of neuroleptics for, 69–73
molindone for, 73
negative symptoms of, 72
overview of neuroleptics for, 5, **6**, **7**, **11**
pimozide for, 3, 69
positive symptoms of, 72
prevalence in children, 5, 67
prevalence of psychotropic drug use for
gender differences in, 29, **30**
related to length of hospitalization, 24–25
psychopharmacological research in children with, 68–69, 74
thioridazine for, 70–73
trifluoperazine for, 71, 72
Schizophreniform disorder, **50**, 56, 61, 72
School refusal, 114, 193–194
Sedation, xx, xxii, 12, 78, 86, 88–89, 99, 107, 114, 126, 143, 146, 162
Sedative-hypnotics, 146
gender differences in use of, **30**
Seizures, 3, 126, 143
Selecting neuroleptics for children, xxi–xxii, 34–35
Self-injurious behavior, 12, 122

Separation anxiety disorder, 114, 161
Serentil. *See* Mesoridazine
Serotonin agonists, 146
Sex hormones, parkinsonism and, 60–61
Sexual abuse, 46, **51**
Sexual dysfunction, 143
Side effects of neuroleptics, xx–xxiii, 43–63, 114, 186. *See also* specific drugs and side effects
  behavioral toxicity, 185–196
  clinicians' fear of inducing, 43, 86
  cognitive effects, 85–114
  criterion symptoms for, **44**
  demographic and behavioral characteristics of subjects evaluated for, 49–50, **50–51**
  gender differences in vulnerability to, 36
  individual case atypicality of tardive dyskinesia and parkinsonism, 44–45, 51, **52–54, 59,** 59–63
    causes of, 59
  methods for study of, 45–49
  noncompliance related to, 15, 37–38, 43
  in patients with tic disorders, 160–163
  related to chlorpromazine-equivalent dose and anticholinergic activity, **52–54,** 55–59
Signal detection theory, 96–98
Simpson Abbreviated Dyskinesia Rating Scale, 46, 76
Sinequan. *See* Doxepin
Sleep disturbances, 194
Social withdrawal, 2, 12, 72, 191, 196
Somnolence, 145
Speech, 87
Stanford Achievement Test, 88
Stealing, 45, **50,** 62, 189, 195
Stelazine. *See* Trifluoperazine
Stereotypies, xx, 2, 12, 121–125
  in children with autism, 122–125
    neuroleptic effects on, 123–125, **124**
    prevalence of, 122
    relation to intelligence, 122–123
    topography of, 123
  clinical conditions associated with, 122
  definition of, 121
  effect of stimulants on, 125
  fenfluramine for, 125
  haloperidol for, 123–125, **124**
  naltrexone for, 125
  rating scales for, 122
  types of, 122
Stimulants
  for attention-deficit/hyperactivity disorder, 32, 139
    with comorbid Tourette's disorder, 156–159
  effect on cognitive tasks, 87, 89–90
  effect on stereotypies, 125
  gender differences in use of, 29, **30**
  for neuroleptic-induced adverse effects, 162
Suicidal ideation, 74, 161, 186, 195
Suicide attempts, 45, **51,** 62, 190, 196
Sulpiride, 145, 180
Symmetrel. *See* Amantadine

Taractan. *See* Chlorprothixene
Tardive dyskinesia, xxiii, 12, 44, 86, 114, 174
  criterion symptoms for, **44**
  effect of anticholinergic treatment on, 62
  estrogens as protection against, 36–37
  evaluation for, 46
  expected responses to changes in medication status, **49**
  individual case atypicality of, 44–45, 51, **52–54,** 59, **59,** 62–63
  methods for study of, 45–49
  prevalence of, 45
    gender differences in, 36–37
    related to length of neuroleptic use, 36
  related to neuroleptic chlorpromazine-equivalent dose and anticholinergic activity, **52–54,** 55–59, 62–63
  risk factors for, 63
Target symptoms, 35
Temper tantrums, 2, 12
Testosterone, 60
Tetrabenazine, for tic disorders, 144
Thiopropazate, for tic disorders, 143
Thioridazine, **6,** 28, 55, 57, 61, 71, 143, 199
  anticholinergic activity factor for, **48**
    paradoxical reaction to, 61
  for attention-deficit/hyperactivity disorder, 3, 32, 98
  chlorpromazine-equivalent dose of, **47**
  cognitive effects of, 88, 98–111. *See also* Cognitive effects
  dosage of, 70, 106
  indications for use in children, 86
  for schizophrenia, 70–73
  for seizures, 3
Thiothixene, 28, 199
  anticholinergic activity factor for, **48**
  for autism, **9**
  chlorpromazine-equivalent dose of, **47**
  dosage of, 70
  for schizophrenia, 5, **10,** 70
Thorazine. *See* Chlorpromazine
Thought disorder, 72, 74, 77, **79,** 83
Tiapride, for tic disorders, 144–145
Tic disorders, 86, 137–164. *See also* Tourette's disorder
  adverse effects of neuroleptics for, 161–163
    behavioral toxicity, 185–196
    cognitive impairment, 161, 171–181
    depression, 161
    dysphoria, 161
    fog states, 86, 147, 162–163
    irritability, 161
    paranoid states, 163
    phobias, 161–162
    stimulants for, 162
  age at onset of, 139
  alpha-methylparatyrosine for, 145
  characteristics of, 138–139
  clinical course of, 151
  clozapine for, 145
  controversial treatments for, 147–148

Tic disorders *(continued)*
definition of tics, 138
diagnosis of, 138–139
disulfiram for, 146
effectiveness of medication for, 139–146
evaluation complicated by spontaneous, nonspecific, and placebo effects, 148–150
fluphenazine for, 142–143, 152–154
haloperidol for, 140–141, 152–154
historical recognition of, 137–138
historical treatments for, 139–140
ineffective treatments for, 146–147
laboratory testing of patient during neuroleptic treatment for, 154–156
metoclopramide for, 144
neuroleptic dosage for, 151–154
not otherwise specified, 138
other phenothiazines for, 143–144
penfluridol for, 142, 154
pimozide for, 141–142, 152–154
piquindone for, 146
predictors of improvement in, 149–150
principles of neuroleptic treatment for, 151–152
prognosis for, 151
recognizing and managing adverse effects of neuroleptics for, 160–163
tetrabenazine for, 144
tiapride for, 144–145
transient versus chronic, 138
treatment indications for, 150–151
treatment regimen for, 152–154
Timed Stereotypies Rating Scale (TSRS), 122
Tindal. *See* Acetophenazine
Toe movements, 122
Tofranil. *See* Imipramine
Tongue discomfort, 78
Tongue movements, 122
Tourette Symptom Global Scale, 175, 177
Tourette's disorder, xx, 2. *See also* Tic disorders
attention-deficit/hyperactivity disorder and, 156–158, 175, 179
use of stimulants for, 156–159
behavioral disorders and, 159–160, 196
clonidine for, 147, 158, 179, 181
cognitive effects of neuroleptics for, 161, 171–181, 186. *See also* Cognitive effects of neuroleptics
diagnosis of, 138
haloperidol for, xxii, xxiii, **9**, 140–141, 172–173
historical recognition of, 137–138
neuroleptic-induced behavioral toxicity in, 185–196
case studies of, 188–195
overview of neuroleptics for, 13
pimozide for, xxii, xxiii, **11**, 12, 141–142, 173

selecting neuroleptics for, xxi–xxiii
treating disorders comorbid with, 156–160
Tourette's Syndrome Severity Scale, 150
Treatment resistance, 35
Tremor, 99
Trifluoperazine, 1–2, **6**, 28, 56–58, 61, 143, 199
anticholinergic activity factor for, **48**
chlorpromazine-equivalent dose of, **47**
for schizophrenia, 71, 72
Trihexyphenidyl, **48**
Trilafon. *See* Perphenazine
L-Tryptophan, 146
Twirling, 122

Valium. *See* Diazepam
Valproic acid, 146
Verapamil, 147
Videotaping of patients, xxiv
Vomiting, 16

Wechsler Intelligence Scale for Children—Revised (WISC-R), 88, 100, **101**
Weight gain, 107, 114, 186, 192
Weight loss, 16
Wide Range Achievement Test, 106
Withdrawal symptoms
dyskinesias, 3, 12, 63, 127, **127**, 174
repeated, 130–132
risk factors for, 130
as indication of noncompliance, 16
Work avoidance, 186